AF345733

Johannes F. Weber

Rediscovering Masculinity

How Natural Remedies Can Improve Your Quality of Life

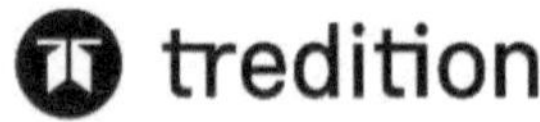

Druck und Distribution im Auftrag des Autors/der Autorin: tredition GmbH, Heinz-Beusen-Stieg 5, 22926 Ahrensburg, Deutschland

Contents

Disclaimer

All of the information contained in this book is presented solely for educational reasons and is not meant to serve as a substitute for professional medical advice or diagnosis. You are alone responsible for determining whether or not you will make use of the natural ingredients described in this book in order to enhance male virility.

The information that is presented in this book is derived from the most recent scientific data and the most up-to-date knowledge that was available at the time of publication. Nevertheless, there is no assurance that the material is correct, comprehensive, or up to date for any reason. In order to make judgments that are based on accurate information, it is the reader's responsibility to review the most recent research and medical literature.

The author and the publisher disclaim any responsibility for any damages, whether direct or indirect, that may be incurred as a consequence of the implementation of the strategies, procedures, or recommendations that are detailed in this book. Each and every reader is strongly urged to seek the advice of a skilled medical professional prior to making use of natural substances or dietary supplements, particularly in the event that they are already experiencing health issues or are on medication.

It is the obligation of the reader to take into consideration the possibility of allergic reactions, intolerances, or combinations with other medications or therapies that may be connected with the utilization of the natural substances that are discussed in this book. Every reader ought to pay close attention to the product labels, dosing instructions, and any potential cautions that are associated with the products that are being used.

The information contained in this book does not constitute a recommendation to buy particular brands or particular goods. Differences may exist in terms of product quality, purity, and production techniques. It is strongly recommended that the reader conduct investigation into the origin, quality, and reliability of the products that were utilized, and if required, seek the opinion of a specialist.

In the end, the reader is the one who is responsible for their own health and how they make use of the natural chemicals that are discussed in this book. Before taking any action based on the information included in this book, each reader should take into consideration his or her particular requirements, medical problems, and personal circumstances, and if required, seek the advice of a practicing physician or other qualified professional.

Introduction

Male virility is a source of power, passion, and vigor for each individual. The beating heart of masculine energy, it has an effect on many aspects of well-being, including self-confidence, relationships, and overall health. There are, however, instances in which male virility can be impacted by elements such as stress, age, or health issues. However, there is no need to be disheartened because nature has a fascinating secret to reveal: twelve natural chemicals that have the ability to retain, increase, and regenerate male vitality like priceless gems.

A mesmerizing voyage into the marvels of nature awaits you in this book, which will take you on a tour across the natural world. We are going to delve deeply into the occurrence, use, origin, and effects of these natural wonders to fully understand them. You are going to experience their strength, uncover their secrets, and enable them to realize their full potential. We will investigate the origins of these drugs and investigate the centuries-old tradition that they have been associated with. Our journey will take us from the wide landscapes of Asia to the exotic regions of South America.

In the course of this excursion, you will gain an understanding of the energizing properties of ginseng, a mysterious root that originates from the Far East. When you are in the Andes, you will be able to inhale the enticing aroma of the maca root and experience the strength that it possesses. As a group, we will investigate the mysterious properties of Yohimbe bark and receive a taste of the wild nature that Africa has to offer. Beginning with Tribulus terrestris and ending with Ashwagandha, we will investigate each of the twelve natural compounds and uncover the distinctive qualities that they possess.

On the other hand, we will not only examine the surface, but we will also delve into the more profound aspects of scientific inquiry. The mechanisms of action of these naturally occurring compounds will be investigated, and we will be able to comprehend the effects that they have on male virility. To accomplish this, we will draw on extensive research in order to provide you with a strong foundation.

It goes without saying that we do not wish to disregard the drawbacks. Because of this, we will take a detailed look at the potential adverse effects that these natural substances may have, and we will also advise you about any potential limitations on their use. Safety and health are of the utmost importance.

The knowledge contained in this book is not the only thing that it contains. This guide is a practical resource that will make it possible for you to include natural substances into your daily life. You are going to discover how to utilize them correctly, how to determine the appropriate dosage, and how to release their maximum potential. We will walk you through the process of utilizing these priceless gifts from nature in order to preserve, enhance, and restore your male virility if you follow our instructions.

We invite you to accompany us on an enthralling excursion across the natural world as we uncover the mysteries of male virility. Allow yourself to be engulfed by the enchantment of nature, and you will find the strength that resides inside you. On the way to a life that is rich in meaning and full of vitality, the book will be your constant companion. Prepared to go on the journey? After that, let us plunge together into the wealth that nature has to offer and the knowledge that its riches possess.

Chapter 1: Ginseng

1.1 History and origin of ginseng

Let's go into the intriguing history of ginseng, a root that has been highly treasured for ages due to the remarkable male virility boosting capabilities it possesses. Ginseng have a long and illustrious cultural past, as they were originally indigenous to the mountainous regions of East Asia. Ginseng was respected as the "root of life" in Korean medicine, while within the context of traditional Chinese medicine, it was referred to as the "king of herbs."

The roots of ginseng have a shape that is similar to that of a human, which is likely one of the reasons for its enormous appeal. Over the course of several centuries, ginseng has been highly regarded for the stimulating and revitalizing effects that it possesses. According to certain accounts, its utilization can be traced back to the first century B.C. Ginseng was regarded by the old wise people as a potentially beneficial source of both physical and mental energy.

Ginseng was not only regarded as a treatment inside East Asian culture, but it was also regarded as a status symbol. Because of its scarcity and the difficulty of cultivating it, it became a product that was in high demand. The pursuit of wild ginseng was frequently regarded as an exciting adventure and was believed to be related with magical ideas. Ginseng hunters were out in the woods, searching for the rare root, hoping for a lucky break that would lead them to it.

These days, ginseng is farmed in a variety of countries, including the United States of America, China, and Korea. There are a few different kinds of ginseng, such as the American ginseng (Panax quinquefolius), the Siberian ginseng (Eleutherococcus senticosus), and the Korean ginseng (Panax ginseng). Traditional medical practices make use of each species for a variety of objectives, and each species possesses its own unique qualities.

The fact that ginseng is not merely a plant but rather a fascinating relationship between man and nature is made abundantly obvious by the fact that its history and cultural importance are so significant. Over the course of the following sections, we will delve more deeply into the many varieties of ginseng and investigate the special potentials that each type possesses for enhancing male virility. Explore the world of ginseng and uncover the wonders that this root has in store for you via your exploration.

1.2 Different types of ginseng and their potential for increasing male virility.

There are variations in the quality of ginseng. In addition to having the ability to improve male virility, this interesting root comes in a variety of various kinds, each of which possesses its own set of distinctive characteristics. In this section, we will take a more in-depth look at the many varieties of ginseng, analyzing their individual qualities as well as the potential for enhancing male vitality.

Among the various species of ginseng, Korean ginseng, also known as Panax ginseng, is likely one of the most well-known and commonly utilized varieties. "True ginseng" is a common name for this herb, which is well-known for the stimulant and adaptogen characteristics that it possesses. Traditionally, Korean ginseng has been utilized for the purpose of enhancing sexual function, mental clarity, and energy levels. In order to improve blood flow and maintain hormonal equilibrium, it has been demonstrated in studies that it can have a beneficial impact on erectile function.

American ginseng, also known as Panax quinquefolius, is a kind of ginseng that is indigenous to North America. It is frequently regarded as a more subdued derivative of Korean ginseng. The effects of this herb are somewhat less intense than those of Korean ginseng, but it is nonetheless utilized for the same purposes. Ginseng from the United States has been shown to improve general health, as well as increase physical stamina and reduce stress. It has the potential to support sexual function and improve libido, both of which are desirable characteristics in male virility.

Eleutherococcus senticosus, sometimes known as Siberian ginseng: Despite the fact that it is not a member of the Panax genus, Siberian ginseng is frequently described to as the "Ginseng of the North." Over the course of history, this adaptogenic herb, which is indigenous to the colder regions of Russia and Asia, has been utilized to improve both physical performance and tolerance to stress. Additionally, Siberian ginseng has the potential to improve male virility by boosting energy levels and enhancing overall well-being.

Ginseng comes in a variety of forms, each of which having its own set of benefits and applications in particular fields. It is essential to keep in mind that the efficacy and virility of different forms of ginseng can depend on a number of different circumstances. These elements include the quality of the product, the appropriate dosage, and the response of the particular body. Therefore, it is recommended that you get ginseng items of a high quality from reliable sources, and if you feel it is required, you should seek the advice of a physician or herbalist in order to make the most appropriate decision for your specific requirements.

Through the acquisition of knowledge regarding the various varieties of ginseng and the comprehension of their capacity to improve male virility, we are able to make use of the numerous treasures that nature provides in order to preserve, enhance, and restore our male vitality. Now that we have a better understanding of the world of ginseng, let's also investigate the interesting roots and unearth the secrets that they conceal.

1.3 Mechanisms of action and scientific findings

Let's take a look behind the curtain and explore the fascinating mechanisms of action of the natural substances that can help increase male virility. Through scientific research and studies, we have gained important insights into how these substances work in the body and what effects they can have on male vitality.

The exact mechanism of action of natural substances is often complex and can vary from substance to substance. In the case of ginseng, for example, it is believed that its active components, such as ginsenosides, can promote blood circulation and influence hormone balance. By improving blood circulation, ginseng may support erectile function. In addition, ginseng is thought to have an adaptogenic effect, meaning that it helps the body cope better with stress, which can have a positive effect on sexual function.

Maca root contains a variety of nutrients such as vitamins, minerals and amino acids. It is believed to balance testosterone production and hormones in the body through its hormonal effects. Through these effects, Maca can increase libido and improve sexual function.

The mode of action of yohimbe bark is based on the active ingredient yohimbine contained in it, which acts as an alpha-2-adrenoceptor antagonist. This can lead to dilation of blood vessels and thus increase blood flow to the genital area. Thus, Yohimbe can be supportive in the treatment of erectile dysfunction.

The exact mechanisms of action of the other natural substances, such as Tribulus terrestris, Ashwagandha or Horny Goat Weed, are also the subject of intensive research. Studies have shown that Tribulus terrestris can increase the production of luteinizing hormone (LH), which can lead to increased testosterone production. Ashwagandha, on the other hand, is believed to balance hormones and protect the body from the effects of stress due to its adaptogenic properties. Horny Goat Weed, due to its association with the active ingredient icariin, is valued for its relaxing effect on smooth muscle and increasing blood supply to the penis.

It is important to note that scientific knowledge on natural substances for male virility is continuously evolving. However, there is already a solid base of research indicating their potential benefits. Nevertheless, it is advisable to wait for further studies and consider the individual body's response.

By understanding the mechanisms of action and scientific findings of the natural substances, we can make informed choices and select those that best suit our individual needs. In the next section, we will look at the proper dosage and possible side effects of these natural substances to ensure safe and effective use.

1.4 Correct dosage and possible side effects

It is essential to determine the appropriate dosage of natural substances for the purpose of enhancing male virility in order to achieve the best possible outcomes and minimize any potential adverse effects. The dosage that is recommended for each chemical can change depending on the specific features of the substance as well as the individual's requirements. Within this section, we will discuss the appropriate dosage for each of the twelve natural ingredients, as well as the potential adverse effects that may be experienced by the individual.

The fact that the dose suggestions in this book are meant to serve as general guidelines should be emphasized on multiple occasions. When it comes to natural chemicals, every body is distinct and may react in a different way. Consequently, before to taking it, it is recommended that you get the advice of a trained medical practitioner or herbalist in order to ascertain the dosage that is suitable for you.

When it comes to ginseng, it is recommended that you take a dosage of approximately 1000 to 2000 milligrams per day in the form of capsules or pills. When increasing the dosage, it is strongly recommended to do so gradually while paying close attention to how the body reacts to the medication. In terms of maca root, the suggested dosage ranges from 1500 to 3000 milligrams per day, with each dose being split into two to three equal portions. In order to ensure that the body is accustomed to the active substances, it is advisable to begin with a smaller dosage and gradually raise it over time.

Because yohimbe bark can be rather powerful, it is important to use caution while determining the appropriate dosage. The normal dosage of yohimbine is between 5 and 15 milligrams per day, which is then divided into two to three doses. It is essential to adhere to the appropriate dosage in order to prevent any potential adverse effects from occurring. The dosage that is recommended for Tribulus terrestris is between 250 and 750 milligrams per day, which should be divided into two to three doses.

When it comes to ashwagandha, the recommended dosage in terms of root extract is between 300 to 500 milligrams per day. To ensure that the active component is distributed evenly throughout the body, it is recommended that the intake be divided into two to three doses. A dosage of 250 to 500 milligrams per day is recommended for the consumption of Horny Goat Weed. This dosage range is determined by the content of the active component icariin.

Taking natural substances might result in adverse effects, particularly if the dosage is incorrect or if an excessive amount is consumed. Headaches, sleep disturbances, and pain in the gastrointestinal tract are some of the potential adverse effects that may be associated with ginseng. Although adverse effects associated with maca root are uncommon, they may include discomfort in the stomach or disruptions in sleep. Yohimbe bark presents a number of potential adverse effects, some of which include elevated blood pressure, palpitations of the heart, and pain in the gastrointestinal tract. Tribulus terrestris is known to have adverse effects that are often moderate and uncommon. Both ashwagandha and horny goat weed are generally well tolerated; nevertheless, certain people may have different sensitivities to them.

It is essential to keep in mind that natural substances as well as other prescriptions can potentially interact with one another. For this reason, it is highly recommended that you see a medical professional prior to using natural substances, particularly if you are already taking conventional medication.

When we utilize the natural ingredients to boost our male virility, we may do so in a way that is both safe and successful if we pay attention to the appropriate amount and take into account any potential adverse effects. For the purpose of making a decision that is both complete and well-informed, let us now delve deeper into the usage restrictions as well as other key features of these natural compounds.

1.5 Restrictions on use and interactions with other drugs

When using natural substances to increase male virility, it is important to consider possible limitations of use and potential interactions with other medications. Each natural substance has its own specific limitations that must be considered to ensure safe and effective use. In this section, we will look at the usage restrictions of the 12 natural substances and provide information on potential interactions with other medications.

With ginseng, use during pregnancy and lactation should be avoided because there is insufficient data on safety. People with certain medical conditions such as high blood pressure, cardiovascular disease, or hormone-dependent cancers should also exercise caution and consult a physician before use. Ginseng may also affect the effects of blood-thinning medications, so monitoring of blood clotting levels may be necessary.

With Maca root, restrictions on use are rare. However, individuals with thyroid problems or hormone-sensitive conditions should be cautious and consult with a physician before use. There are reports of interactions with certain medications, such as those used to treat thyroid disorders, and it is recommended to discuss these with a physician.

Yohimbe bark may have strong interactions with various medications. People with heart problems, high blood pressure, liver disease or mental disorders should avoid yohimbe. There is also a possibility of interactions with antidepressants, antihypertensive drugs, and other medications. Careful consideration of the risks and benefits and medical advice are essential in this case.

With Tribulus terrestris, use restrictions are generally low, but people with hormone-sensitive conditions should exercise caution and consult a physician before use. Ashwagandha is generally well tolerated, but people with autoimmune disorders or hormone-sensitive conditions should consult a physician before use. Horny Goat Weed should be avoided by people with heart disease or low blood pressure.

It is important to note that natural substances may also interact with other medications. Ginseng may affect the effects of blood thinning medications, while maca root and yohimbe bark may potentially affect the effects of certain medications. It is highly recommended to talk to a doctor about possible interactions before using natural substances, especially if you are already taking medications.

By following the usage restrictions and possible interactions with other medications, we can safely and effectively use the natural substances to increase our male virility. In the next section, we will talk about other important aspects, such as the proper storage and shelf life of the natural substances, to ensure that we can use their full potential.When considering the use of natural substances to enhance male virility, it is essential to take into consideration the potential potential for interactions with other medications as well as the possible limitations of use. In order to ensure that the use of natural substances is both safe and effective, it is necessary to take into consideration the specific limits that are associated with each natural material. In this section, we will discuss the limitations of the twelve natural compounds. Additionally, we will provide information on the possible interactions that these substances may have with other pharmaceuticals.

When it comes to ginseng, it is best to avoid using it during pregnancy and lactation because there is not enough information available regarding its safety. Additionally, individuals who suffer from specific medical disorders, such as high blood pressure, cardiovascular disease, or tumors that are dependent on hormones, should exercise caution and seek the advice of a physician prior to using the product. In addition, ginseng has the potential to influence the effects of medications that thin the blood; hence, it is essential to check the levels of blood clotting.

There are very few restrictions placed on the use of maca root. On the other hand, people who have thyroid issues or diseases that are sensitive to hormones have to exercise caution and seek the advice of a medical professional before using this product. Certain drugs, such as those used to treat thyroid issues, have been shown to have interactions with other medications; therefore, it is important that you discuss these interactions with a medical professional.

There are a number of drugs that may have significant interactions with yohimbe bark. Yohimbe should be avoided by individuals who suffer from diseases related to the heart, high blood pressure, liver illness, or mental disorders. It is also possible for this medication to interact negatively with other prescriptions, such as antidepressants, antihypertensive meds, and other pharmaceuticals. This situation calls for careful assessment of the potential hazards and advantages, as well as the counsel of a medical professional.

In general, there are not many restrictions placed on the usage of Tribulus terrestris; nevertheless, individuals who have conditions that are sensitive to hormones should exercise caution and seek the advice of a physician before using it. In most cases, ashwagandha is well tolerated; nevertheless, individuals who suffer from autoimmune disorders or ailments that are sensitive to hormones should seek medical advice prior to using this herb. Individuals who suffer from cardiovascular disease or have low blood pressure should steer clear of horny goat weed.

It is essential to keep in mind that natural substances as well as other prescriptions can potentially interact with one another. Ginseng has the ability to influence the effects of blood-thinning drugs, whereas maca root and yohimbe bark have the capacity to influence the effects of some pharmaceuticals for the same reason. Before beginning to use natural substances, it is strongly advised that you see a medical professional about the potential combinations of these substances, particularly if you are already taking medication.

It is feasible for us to boost our male virility in a way that is both safe and effective by using natural drugs, provided that we adhere to the usage restrictions and consider the potential interactions with other treatments. When we move on to the following section, we will discuss further significant elements, such as the appropriate storage and shelf life of the natural ingredients, in order to guarantee that we are able to make full use of their potential.

Chapter 2: Maca root

2.1 Origin and cultural significance of the Maca root

Maca root is a natural ingredient that has been treasured for its virility-enhancing properties for a very long time. Join us on this intriguing journey to the Maca root. The high altitudes of the Andes in Peru are the source of maca root, which has been farmed and utilized by the indigenous people of the region for generations already. In addition to having a deep cultural importance for the indigenous peoples of the region, it is frequently referred to as "Peruvian ginseng."

The maca root is considered a holy gift from the natural world by the indigenous people who live in the Andes. As a representation of fecundity, strength, and perseverance, they hold it in high esteem. The maca plant, from which the root is harvested, is able to grow in harsh environments at elevations of up to 4,000 meters above sea level. In these environments, the plant must be able to survive strong winds, intense sunlight, and extreme temperatures. These unfavorable conditions are what endow the maca root with its remarkable qualities and elevate it to the status of a genuine gem.

Vitamins, minerals, amino acids, and plant sterols are only some of the components that are found in maca root, which has a distinctive composition. The virility-enhancing qualities of maca root are attributed to the particular combination of chemicals that it contains. For centuries, people have used it to boost their libido, enhance their sexual performance, and improve their overall health and well-being.

The root of the maca plant has an adaptogenic effect, which implies that it assists the body in better adjusting to difficult times and circumstances. The production of sex hormones, including testosterone, can be influenced by it, and it can also help to maintain hormonal balance. Increasing sexual desire, improving sexual function, and increasing general vitality and stamina are all possible outcomes that can be attributed to the effects of maca root.

Not only is the root of the maca plant grown and consumed in Peru these days, but it is also consumed in other areas of the world. This substance can be obtained in a number of different forms, such as powder, capsules, and extract. In order to achieve the greatest possible outcomes, it is essential to purchase Maca goods of a significant quality from reliable providers.

It is abundantly obvious that maca root is not only a natural material, but also a symbol of vigor and fertility, as evidenced by the rich history of maca root and the cultural significance of maca root. As we progress through the following sections, we will delve deeper into the characteristics and applications of maca root in order to have a better understanding of its full potential for enhancing male vitality. Exploring the world of maca root and learning about the incredible benefits it may provide for you is an awesome experience.

2.2 Nutrient content and potential benefits for male virility

Not only is the maca root notable for its cultural significance, but it is also remarkable for the excellent nutrient content that it possesses, which may provide significant benefits for male virility concerns. The root contains a wide variety of nutrients that are necessary for maintaining good sexual function as well as overall vitality of the body. We are going to take a more in-depth look at the nutrient content of maca root as well as the potential benefits that it may have for male virility in this part.

The maca root includes a number of different vitamins, including vitamins C, E, and B vitamins, all of which play a significant part in the production of energy and the maintenance of a healthy hormone balance. These vitamins are beneficial to the healthy functioning of sexual organs and contribute to the overall health of the reproductive system.

Additionally, maca root contains a high concentration of minerals, including calcium, magnesium, zinc, and iron. The creation of sex hormones and the maintenance of a healthy libido both require these minerals, which are essential for proper functioning. Zinc plays a particularly significant role in male virility since it helps to increase the synthesis of testosterone and has the potential to improve the effectiveness of sperm.

It is also possible to find amino acids in maca root, which are the fundamental components of protein. The creation of neurotransmitters, which are essential for sexual arousal and mood in general, is dependent on these amino acids, which play a significant role in the process. Maca root contains a number of amino acids, including arginine and histidine, which have the ability to enhance blood flow, which in turn can contribute to an improvement in erection quality.

In addition, maca root includes plant sterols, which are pre-hormones that are necessary for the formation of sex hormones. These sterols have the ability to maintain hormonal equilibrium, which in turn helps to support male virility. Additionally, maca root includes phytochemicals such as glucosinolates and flavonoids, which have the potential to have anti-inflammatory and antioxidant activities.

Maca root is a natural material that has the potential to increase male virility due to the combination of these nutrients being present in it. By boosting a healthy libido, enhancing blood flow, and supporting a healthy hormone balance, maca root has the potential to assist in the enhancement of sexual function and general well-being.

It is essential to keep in mind that the repercussions of maca root can differ from person to person. While some men may have a more rapid improvement in their virility, others may experience a more gradual change. In order to achieve the best possible outcomes, it is advocated that maca root be consumed over an extended period of time.

In order to ensure that you get the most out of this natural material, we will discuss the various kinds of maca root as well as the recommended dosages in the following sections. Gain an understanding of the natural power of maca root and how it can enhance the vitality of your male body.

2.3 Different forms of application (powders, capsules, extracts)

Maca root is commercially available in a variety of forms, which enables us to include it into our daily routine in a variety of different ways. Because every type of application comes with its own set of benefits and drawbacks, it is essential that we select the one that caters to our specific requirements in the most effective manner. In this part of the article, we will discuss the various ways in which maca root can be applied, such as powders, capsules, and extracts.

Among the several ways that maca can be applied, powder is among the most typical. It is prepared from maca roots that have been dried and crushed, and it may be readily mixed into a variety of dishes and beverages, including cereals, yogurt, smoothies, and beverages. The powder has a flavor that is not overpowering and goes well with a wide variety of flavors. Different people have different require-ments, thus the dosage of the powder can be altered accordingly. In order to ensure that the body is ac-customed to the active substances, it is advisable to begin with a smaller dosage and gradually raise it over time.

Taking maca root in the form of capsules is a con-venient and practical method of consumption. All of the root powder is contained within capsules that are designed to be readily ingested. Due to the fact that the dosage is already predetermined in the cap-sules, correct dosing is permitted. Those individuals who desire exact control over dosage will find this to be an exceptionally convenient option. You can easily incorporate the capsules into your regular supplement routine, and they are perfect for taking with you when you are on the road.

Maca extracts are forms of the maca root that are extremely concentrated and contain a greater quantity of active components than other forms would. They are often sold in liquid form, and they can be consumed on their own or mixed into beverages like soda or water. Due to the fact that the dosage of the extracts might change based on the concentration, it is essential to adhere to the dosage guidelines provided by the manufacturer. The extracts provide a quick and effective absorption of the active components, making them an excellent choice for individuals who favor a form of Maca root that is relatively high in concentration.

If you want to select the most appropriate form of maca root application, it is essential to take into consideration your own preferences and requirements. People who desire the ability to integrate powder into a variety of various recipes will find powder to be beneficial. For people who seek precise dose and want to simplify their intake, capsules are an excellent choice. The absorption of the active substances is facilitated by extracts in a quick and effective manner.

It is essential to only purchase Maca goods of the highest possible quality from reputable suppliers, regardless of the manner in which you intend to utilize it. To guarantee that you get the most out of the maca root, you should look for a product that is of high quality, pure, and can be traced back to its origin.

In the next part, we will discuss the right dosages of maca root in order to guarantee that we make the most of the possible benefits that it may have for male virility. Let us delve deeper into the interesting world of maca root and uncover the astonishing impacts that it has on our energy.

2.4 Studies and clinical research results

The usefulness of maca root in enhancing male virility has been the subject of investigation in a number of investigations and clinical research projects. A significant amount of information regarding the possible advantages and mechanisms of action of maca root is provided by these studies. In the next section, we will examine a few of these studies as well as the findings that were obtained from the research.

An investigation on the impact that Maca has on sexual function was carried out in a clinical research with male participants. Participants who took Maca for a period of twelve weeks reported a significant improvement in their sexual desire and pleasure when compared to the group that received a placebo. Maca may boost sexual performance by increasing libido and improving erectile function, according to the findings of the study.

In another study, the effects of Maca on the quality of sperm in males who had reproductive needs that were not being addressed were explored. It was shown that ingesting Maca for a period of four months led to a considerable improvement in sperm count, motility, and morphology. The results showed that this improvement was meaningful. Based on these findings, it appears that Maca may have a beneficial effect on testosterone levels in males.

Furthermore, a number of in vitro experiments have been conducted to study the bioactive chemicals that are found in maca root. According to the findings of these investigations, specific components found in maca root have the potential to have a beneficial impact on the regulation of hormones, particularly with regard to the creation of testosterone. It is also possible that they possess anti-inflammatory and antioxidant effects, both of which are beneficial to one's overall health.

Despite the fact that these studies have produced encouraging findings, it is essential to emphasize that additional study is required in order to comprehend the precise mechanisms of action of maca root and to validate its safety and effectiveness over an extended period of treatment. There is a wide range of possible outcomes since the active components found in maca root are absorbed by the body in a manner that is unique to each individual.

It is also essential to keep in mind that natural compounds like maca root are typically regarded as dietary supplements and are not authorized for use as drugs for the treatment of medical diseases. Maca root should not be considered the only solution to sexual difficulties or health conditions; rather, it should be considered as part of a balanced lifestyle and nutrition.

In the following part, we will discuss the potential use restrictions and measures that should be taken when utilizing Maca root in order to guarantee that we are utilizing it in a responsible and safe manner. Proceed with your exploration of the fascinating world of natural substances and learn about the numerous methods in which you can enhance your male vitality.

2.5 Safety profiles and possible contraindications

As long as it is consumed in the recommended quantities, maca root is usually considered to be safe. However, in order to guarantee that the use of the product is safe, it is necessary to take into consideration specific safety profiles and potential contraindications. Within the scope of this part, we will investigate the safety profile of maca root and the potential contraindications that may be associated with its use.

The majority of people have no adverse reactions to maca root. Side effects are uncommon, but they can happen under certain circumstances. These include discomfort in the stomach, issues with the digestive system, or moderate abnormalities in sleep. Typically, these adverse effects are not severe and don't last long. It is recommended that the amount of maca root taken be decreased or stopped entirely if these negative effects occur.

It is important to show caution while dealing with certain demographics in particular. It is recommended that women who are pregnant or breastfeeding refrain from using maca root preparations because there is little knowledge regarding the effects of these preparations on pregnancy and breastfeeding. It is strongly suggested that you select other natural substances or seek the advice of a medical professional during these occasions.

It is especially important for individuals who have hormone-sensitive diseases, such as breast or prostate cancer, to take caution and seek the advice of a medical professional before consuming Maca products. Considering that there are some findings that show Maca can impact the balance of hormones, it is essential to take this into consideration while dealing with specific conditions that are sensitive to hormones.

On top of that, maca root might have an effect on the way certain medications work. Before beginning to use maca root, you should consider the possibility of drug interactions with your physician if you are currently taking any medications by consulting with them. Medications that are used to treat thyroid diseases, blood pressure difficulties, or hormone imbalances are particularly susceptible to this phenomenon (especially).

There are no particular medical claims that can be made regarding maca root because it is considered a nutritional supplement. This is a crucial point to keep in mind. Maca root should not be considered the only solution to sexual difficulties or health conditions; rather, it should be considered as part of a balanced lifestyle and nutrition.

As a result of the fact that every person reacts differently to maca root, it is essential to pay attention to your own requirements and recognize any potential contraindications. Seek the advice of a medical professional if you have any concerns or specific health conditions.

In the following section, we will discuss the appropriate dosage of maca root in order to ensure that we gain the maximum benefit from the possible advantages that it offers for enhancing male vitality. Learn about the natural power of maca root and how it can improve your sexual health as well as your quality of life in general.

Chapter 3: Yohimbe bark

3.1 History and geographical distribution of the yohimbe tree

Yohimbe bark is a natural ingredient that has been treasured for its virility-enhancing powers for a very long time. Join us on this intriguing journey to the yohimbe bark. Pausinystalia yohimbe, more commonly referred to as the Yohimbe tree, is a species of evergreen tree that is indigenous to the tropical rainforests of West Africa. There is a strong connection between the indigenous peoples of Africa and the yohimbe tree, which has a rich and varied history that dates back to ancient times.

The bark of the Yohimbe tree has been utilized by African tribes for ages as a cure and aphrodisiac. Yohimbe trees are native to Africa. According to their beliefs, the yohimbe bark contributes to an increase in sexual virility and libido. Both the tree and its bark hold significant cultural meanings and are frequently utilized in the ceremonies and rituals that are performed in Africa.

It is in the humid rainforest regions of West Africa, specifically in nations like Nigeria, Cameroon, Gabon, and the Congo, that the yohimbe tree may be found growing. It has the ability to grow to a height of up to thirty meters, and the bark of the tree is a distinctive reddish-brown color. Yohimbine, which is recognized for its ability to increase virility, is found in the bark of the yohimbe tree. Yohimbine is the active ingredient.

The traditional application of yohimbe bark to enhance male virility has resulted in the bark's growing popularity in other regions of the world during the past several decades. In modern times, yohimbe bark can be purchased in a variety of forms, including powder, capsules, and extracts alike.

The usage of yohimbe bark, on the other hand, calls for extra caution and responsible behavior because of the potentially powerful effects it possesses. It is essential to ensure that the dosage and monitoring are correct in order to reduce the likelihood of experiencing any adverse effects.

The yohimbe tree is not only a natural substance, but it also has a cultural value and tradition in Africa, as evidenced by its intriguing history and geographical distribution. This is made evident by the fact that the yohimbe tree is indigenous to Africa. As we progress through the following sections, we will delve deeper into the characteristics and applications of Yohimbe bark in order to gain a better understanding of its entire potential for enhancing male vitality. Discover the remarkable advantages that the Yohimbe tree has to offer you by delving into its habitat and learning about its benefits.

3.2 Active ingredients and their influence on male virility

There are a variety of active components found in yohimbe bark, and these components have the potential to influence male virility. Yohimbine, an alkaloid that functions as a natural stimulant and has the ability to increase blood flow, is the most important active element this product contains. The usage of this active ingredient to enhance sexual function and libido has been documented for a significant amount of time.

The action of yohimbine is to inhibit the adrenaline receptors, which in turn causes an increase in the amount of nitric oxide that is released. One of the chemical compounds known as nitric oxide is a vasodilator, which means that it causes blood vessels to expand. The increase in blood flow to the vaginal region that results from this dilatation can potentially result in an enhanced erection.

In addition, yohimbine has the ability to stimulate the release of norepinephrine, which is a neurotransmitter that has an effect on sexual arousal and libido expression. The release of more norepinephrine may contribute to an increase in sexual desire and contribute to an improvement in sexual function.

The effect that yohimbine has on male virility might differ from person to person, which is a crucial fact to keep in mind. It is possible that the effect will be more pronounced in some guys than it will be in others, and it is also likely that not every man will perceive the same reaction. In order to obtain the desired benefits and reduce the likelihood of experiencing any adverse effects, the ideal dosage should be properly measured and weighed.

Additionally to yohimbine, the bark of the yohimbe tree includes a number of additional alkaloids and active chemicals, including johimban, corynanthidine, and corynoxein-like substances. Despite the fact that the precise mechanisms underlying these substances are not yet completely understood, it is possible that they may contribute to the virility-enhancing effect. All of these active components work together to promote sexual function and may also contribute to an increase in male virility by themselves.

At the same time, it is essential to stress that the use of yohimbe bark has to be carried out with caution and in the proper quantities. Inappropriately high doses of yohimbine have the potential to bring about unfavorable side effects, including elevated blood pressure, a rapid heartbeat, nausea, and dizziness. For this reason, it is highly recommended that you consult with a medical professional before beginning to consume yohimbe products, particularly if you are currently on medication or have any pre-existing health conditions.

To ensure that you are able to use Yohimbe bark in a manner that is both safe and successful, we will examine the various methods in which it can be utilized in the next section. Become familiar with the remarkable properties of Yohimbe Bark and the ways in which it can enhance your male vitality.There are a variety of active components found in yohimbe bark, and these components have the potential to influence male virility. Yohimbine, an alkaloid that functions as a natural stimulant and has the ability to increase blood flow, is the most important active element this product contains. The usage of this active ingredient to enhance sexual function and libido has been documented for a significant amount of time.

The action of yohimbine is to inhibit the adrenaline receptors, which in turn causes an increase in the amount of nitric oxide that is released. One of the chemical compounds known as nitric oxide is a vasodilator, which means that it causes blood vessels to expand. The increase in blood flow to the vaginal region that results from this dilatation can potentially result in an enhanced erection.

In addition, yohimbine has the ability to stimulate the release of norepinephrine, which is a neurotransmitter that has an effect on sexual arousal and libido expression. The release of more norepinephrine may contribute to an increase in sexual desire and contribute to an improvement in sexual function.

The effect that yohimbine has on male virility might differ from person to person, which is a crucial fact to keep in mind. It is possible that the effect will be more pronounced in some guys than it will be in others, and it is also likely that not every man will perceive the same reaction. In order to obtain the desired benefits and reduce the likelihood of experiencing any adverse effects, the ideal dosage should be properly measured and weighed.

Additionally to yohimbine, the bark of the yohimbe tree includes a number of additional alkaloids and active chemicals, including johimban, corynanthidine, and corynoxein-like substances. Despite the fact that the precise mechanisms underlying these substances are not yet completely understood, it is possible that they may contribute to the virility-enhancing effect. All of these active components work together to promote sexual function and may also contribute to an increase in male virility by themselves.

At the same time, it is essential to stress that the use of yohimbe bark has to be carried out with caution and in the proper quantities. Inappropriately high doses of yohimbine have the potential to bring about unfavorable side effects, including elevated blood pressure, a rapid heartbeat, nausea, and dizziness. For this reason, it is highly recommended that you consult with a medical professional before beginning to consume yohimbe products, particularly if you are currently on medication or have any pre-existing health conditions.

To ensure that you are able to use Yohimbe bark in a manner that is both safe and successful, we will examine the various methods in which it can be utilized in the next section. Become familiar with the remarkable properties of Yohimbe Bark and the ways in which it can enhance your male vitality.

3.3 Possible applications and suitable dosages

When it comes to taking use of the virility-enhancing effects of yohimbe bark, it can be applied in a variety of different forms. There are a few different ways to consume the bark, and maintaining the appropriate dosage is of the utmost importance. In this part of the article, we will discuss the various uses that Yohimbe bark can be used for, as well as the dosages that are recommended.

It is common practice to sell yohimbe bark in the form of an extract or powder. When utilizing the extract, it is essential to cautiously adhere to the dosage recommendations provided by the extract's manufacturer. Due to the fact that the dosage may change based on the concentration of the extract, it is essential to ensure that the amount that is advised is not exceeded. In order to determine an individual's level of tolerance, it is advisable to begin with a lower dosage and progressively raise it over time.

On the off chance that you want to make use of yohimbe powder, you can put it to a number of different uses. As an illustration, you may put the powder inside capsules and then consume it through the mouth. It is essential to carry out precise measurements of the dosage and to avoid exceeding the amount that is suggested. Alternatively, the powder can be mixed with liquids like water or juice and then consumed. This is another option. The exact dosage is determined by the individual's tolerance level and the results that are desired.

Yohimbe bark, on the other hand, has the potential to produce significant effects, which is a crucial point to keep in mind. As a result, it is recommended to give careful consideration to the dosage and to avoid taking quantities that are excessive. Yohimbine can cause undesirable side effects if it is used in excessive amounts, including a rise in blood pressure, a rapid heartbeat, and unpleasant feelings of nausea. It is recommended that you get the advice of a medical professional prior to utilizing yohimbe bark if you have any worries or pre-existing health disorders.

Noting that the effects of Yohimbe bark can differ from person to person is another crucial point to keep in mind. There is a possibility that the results will differ from one individual to the next, and not every man experiences the same reaction. The full effects of Yohimbe bark might not be experienced for a while, depending on the individual. If you want to evaluate the benefits of the virility-enhancing substance, it is recommended that you continue using it for a decent amount of time.

For the purpose of ensuring the purity and quality of the bark, it is recommended to select yohimbe goods of a high grade from manufacturers recognized for their reliability. This is of utmost importance in order to guarantee that you achieve the desired outcomes and reduce the likelihood of any potential risks.

As we move on to the following part, we will discuss the potential risks and contraindications associated with the utilization of yohimbe bark. We are going to go deeper into the world of natural compounds and find out how these substances can naturally improve your male vitality.

3.4 Adverse reactions and precautions

The utilization of Yohimbe bark as a means to enhance male virility may be associated with the possibility of undesirable side effects. It is essential to be aware of these adverse effects and to take the necessary precautions in order to carry out the use in a safe manner. In the next section, we will discuss the possible adverse effects as well as the essential measures to take.

The consumption of Yohimbe bark may result in adverse effects for certain persons. There is a wide range of possible variations from person to person, and not all users exhibit these characteristics. Increased blood pressure, a faster heartbeat, dizziness, nausea, and anxiousness are some of the undesirable side effects that may occur. It is essential to keep a close eye out for these allergic responses and to limit or stop using Yohimbe bark if any of these adverse effects manifest themselves.

There are also particular groups of people for whom it is recommended to use caution. It is recommended that individuals who already have cardiovascular disease, excessive blood pressure, or cardiac arrhythmias refrain from consuming yohimbe bark or seek the advice of a medical professional before commencing its use. These diseases may become even more severe as a result of the bark's stimulating effect on circulation, which may also result in complications that are not ideal.

In addition, individuals who suffer from liver disease, kidney issues, or gastrointestinal disorders have to take caution as well. The function of these organs can be negatively impacted by yohimbe bark, which can also lead to difficulties. It is recommended to seek medical advice in advance in order to explain any potential hazards.

Remember that the effect of yohimbe bark may interact with the effects of other medications or dietary supplements. This is a crucial point to keep in mind. To be more specific, the usage of yohimbe bark in conjunction with specific drugs for the treatment of hypertension, heart problems, or mental disease may result in interactions that are not ideal. Therefore, before to consuming Yohimbe bark, it is recommended to check with a medical professional in order to take into consideration any potential interactions or contraindications.

It is not recommended that women who are pregnant or breastfeeding use yohimbe bark because there is insufficient knowledge regarding the safety of the substance and its effects on the developing child or fetus. During these period of time, it is essential to select alternative natural substances or to seek the advice of a medical professional.

In conclusion, it is recommended to obtain yohimbe goods of a high quality from reputable manufacturers in order to guarantee the purity and quality of the bark. In order to reduce the likelihood of experiencing any adverse effects, it is essential to adhere to the dosage that has been suggested.

As we move on to the following part, we will discuss the limitations of yohimbe bark's application as well as the potential interactions it may have with other medicines and medications. Discover how to utilize yohimbe bark in a way that is both safe and effective in order to boost your male vitality and have a sexual life that is more satisfying.

3.5 Legal aspects and availability of yohimbe products

Whenever you use items containing yohimbe, it is essential to take into consideration the legal implications and the accessibility of these products. As a result of the fact that yohimbe bark has the ability to increase virility, it is subject to particular legal laws and limits in certain countries. For the purpose of this part, we shall discuss the legal implications of yohimbe products as well as their availability.

It's possible that the legal status surrounding yohimbe will be different in each new country. Yohimbe products are subject to stringent regulations in certain countries, and in order to purchase or use them, one must have the required authorization or a prescription from a medical professional. When considering the purchase or use of yohimbe items, it is essential to acquire knowledge regarding the legal framework that governs your country.

The nutritional supplement known as yohimbe is accessible for purchase in certain countries, and it does not require a prescription from a medical practitioner. In situations like these, it is still a good idea to evaluate the quality of the items and buy yohimbe products that are of a high quality from producers that you consider to be reliable.

When purchasing items containing yohimbe, it is essential to pay close attention to the correct labeling and the components that are included. Manufacturers who can be trusted provide information that is easy to understand on dose, ingredients, and the instructions for suggested usage. For the purpose of ensuring the efficacy and purity of yohimbe products, it is advisable to select goods that are created in accordance with stringent quality requirements.

Yohimbe products might not be available in all nations or locations, which is another thing that should be taken into consideration. There may be variations in availability as a result of regulatory regulations and the demand that varies across different markets. In the event that yohimbe products are not readily available or do not satisfy individual requirements, it may be essential to search for alternatives or to make use of other natural compounds in order to boost male virility.

In conclusion, before to utilizing Yohimbe products, it is recommended that you examine the legal framework in your country and ensure that you are obtaining items of a high quality from producers that you can rely on. It is important to ensure that you follow the dose guidelines and precautions.

We are going to take a closer look at the origin of this natural material as well as its virility-enhancing properties in the following chapter. This natural ingredient is another one that has been shown to increase male virility. Discover how natural substances can help your male vitality in a way that is both natural and effective by delving into the world of natural substances.

Chapter 4: Tribulus terrestris

4.1 Botanical characteristics and natural occurrence of Tribulus terrestris

The plant species known as Tribulus terrestris, which is often referred to as earth burr thorn or earth star, is a member of the family of plants known as yokelets. A number of regions around the world, including Europe, Asia, Africa, and Australia, are characterized by its prevalence. Deserts, savannas, and stony soils are the ideal environments for the growth of Tribulus terrestris, which thrives in dry and warm environments.

Plants belonging to the genus Tribulus are distinguished by their little yellow flowers and thorny fruits, both of which are distinctive of the plant class. When the fruits are touched, they might hook on the skin due to their hardness and the sharp thorns that they contain. The name "Burzel thorn" was given to the plant as a result of this characteristic.

Tribulus terrestris has been utilized for a considerable amount of time in a variety of complementary and alternative medicine practices, such as Ayurvedic medicine and Chinese medicine. It is very important to cherish the fruits and other portions of the plant that are above ground because of the virility-enhancing and health-promoting properties that they possess.

The plant is known to contain a variety of bioactive chemicals, such as steroids, flavonoids, and so-called saponins. Currently, these substances are being investigated for the possible impact that they may have on the sexual health and virility of men.

Tribulus terrestris is frequently regarded as a natural aphrodisiac by many people since it has the ability to boost sexual desire and performance in males. The bioactive components found in the plant are thought to be responsible for the increased synthesis of nitric oxide, which in turn can result in an increase in the amount of blood that flows to the genital region. The enhancement of blood flow may, in turn, lead to the enhancement of erectile function and strength of sexual desire.

When it comes to the impact that Tribulus terrestris has on male virility, the scientific evidence is contradictory, which is a crucial point to keep in mind. Although some studies have revealed that there is a favorable influence on sexual function, other studies have not discovered any meaningful effects for sexual function. There is a possibility that the effects of Tribulus terrestris could differ from person to person and depend on other factors such as lifestyle and general health.

In the following chapter, we will examine the scientific evidence that supports the virility-enhancing characteristics of Tribulus terrestris and take a more in-depth look at these properties. Explore the ways in which this natural substance can help you maintain your male vitality, as well as the various ways in which it can be utilized to attain the outcomes you seek.

4.2 Link between Tribulus terrestris and male virility

It has been known for a long time that Tribulus terrestris is related with male virility and is thought to be a drug that enhances virility. In this section, we shall investigate the relationship between Tribulus terrestris and male virility in further detail.

Tribulus terrestris has been shown to have a number of different explanations for its virility-enhancing qualities. The presence of bioactive chemicals, particularly those that are referred to as saponins, within the plant is one hypothesis that could be considered. The presence of these saponins may be responsible for the elevation of testosterone levels, which may, in turn, have a beneficial effect on the virility of males. When it comes to men's sexual function and libido, testosterone is an essential hormone on the list.

Furthermore, it is suspected that Tribulus terrestris can enhance the circulation of blood to the vaginal region. In order to maintain a good erection and sexual performance, it is essential to have better blood flow. Tribulus terrestris may help widen blood vessels, which in turn improves blood flow to the penis. This is accomplished by boosting nitric oxide levels.

There is a lack of consensus among researchers on the relationship between Tribulus terrestris and male virility, which is a crucial point to keep in mind. A number of studies have demonstrated favorable outcomes, indicating that men who took Tribulus terrestris saw an enhancement in their sexual function as well as an increase in their testosterone levels. Other research, on the other hand, has not been able to uncover any substantial consequences. It is likely that the effects of Tribulus terrestris could differ from one person to the next and depend on a variety of factors including overall health, hormone levels, and dose. Both of these elements are important considerations.

In addition, it is essential to emphasize that Tribulus terrestris should not be seen as a miracle cure for sexual issues. While it is a natural drug that has the potential to be supportive, it cannot be the only solution to sexual issues that are more complex. If you want to attain the best possible outcomes, it might be beneficial to utilize Tribulus terrestris in conjunction with a healthy lifestyle, a balanced diet, and frequent physical activity.

We are going to take a more in-depth look at the findings and research that have been conducted in the scientific community regarding the connection between Tribulus terrestris and male virility in this chapter. In order to offer you with an informed decision-making basis for utilizing this natural substance to enhance your male vitality, we will also discuss the many applications of Tribulus terrestris as well as the dosages that are recommended for those applications.

4.3 Effects on hormone balance and sexual function

There is a common association between Tribulus terrestris and impacts on hormone balance and sexual function. This is because of the virility-enhancing characteristics that it possesses. Within this section, we will delve more into the impact that Tribulus terrestris has on the hormonal equilibrium as well as the functioning of the sexual organs.

One of the potential effects that Tribulus terrestris may have on the equilibrium of hormones is the possibility of a rise in testosterone levels. The primary male sex hormone, testosterone, is associated with the maintenance of sexual function, libido, and overall vigor. It plays a significant role in these relationships. It has been demonstrated through research that the consumption of Tribulus terrestris can lead to a rise in testosterone levels, which in turn can have a beneficial impact on sexual function.

Additionally, it is believed that Tribulus terrestris can enhance the amount of nitric oxide that is released. The relaxing of blood vessels is facilitated by a chemical component known as nitric oxide, which plays an important part in the process. It is possible that increased blood flow will result in improved erectile function, which will in turn support sexual function.

Take notice that the effects of Tribulus terrestris on hormone balance and sexual function may vary depending on a number of different conditions. This is a crucial point to keep in mind. In this context, "individual response" refers to factors such as dosage and length of usage, as well as general health and other factors that may contribute to sexual issues. Before beginning to use Tribulus terrestris, it is strongly suggested that you get the advice of a medical professional or an expert, particularly in the event that you have a history of hormone imbalances or sexual issues.

In addition, it is essential to keep in mind that Tribulus terrestris is offered as a dietary supplement; however, it should not be regarded as a replacement for a well-balanced diet and a healthy way of life. Maintaining healthy sexual function requires a number of critical elements, including a nutritious diet, participating in regular physical activity, and getting enough sleep.

Throughout the course of this chapter, we will investigate in great detail the effects that Tribulus terrestris has on the hormonal equilibrium and sexual function. The purpose of this presentation is to give you with an informed basis for decision-making by presenting scientific facts and studies. Note, however, that individual outcomes may vary, and it is recommended that you seek the opinion of a specialist if you feel that you require it.

4.4 Recommended dosages and duration of use

Tribulus terrestris should be used for the appropriate amount of time and at the appropriate dosage in order to achieve the best possible outcomes and reduce the likelihood of any adverse effects. In the next part, we will discuss the dosages that are recommended as well as the period of use for Tribulus terrestris.

The fact that there is no one suggestion for the dosage of Tribulus terrestris is an essential point to keep in mind. This is because there are many different elements that need to be taken into consideration, such as the product, the concentration of bioactive ingredients, and individual variances. The instructions that are printed on the product label should be followed, or you should seek the advice of a medical professional or other knowledgeable individual.

In most cases, the suggested daily dosage ranges from 250 to 1500 milligrams. It is possible to divide these dosages into two or three single doses and spread them out throughout the day. To assess the patient's tolerance and reduce the likelihood of experiencing adverse effects, it may be recommended to begin with a lower dosage. It is possible to make the necessary adjustments to the dosage over time in order to get the desired results.

It is also possible for the length of use of Tribulus terrestris to vary. After observing the consumption for a period of time ranging from four to eight weeks, it is advisable to analyze the effect. There is evidence from a few research that suggests that after this period of time, there may be good impacts on sexual function and hormone balance. There is also the possibility of using it for a longer period of time;

however, this should be done in collaboration with a medical professional or an expert.

It is essential to ensure that the dosages and duration of use are not exceeded beyond what is indicated. It is possible that excessive use of Tribulus terrestris could result in unfavorable side effects and raise the risk of associated issues. If you have any queries regarding the dosage or the length of time you should use the product, it is best to seek the counsel of a specialist.

In addition, it is essential to emphasize that Tribulus terrestris should not be seen as a long-term cure to sexual issues. Despite the fact that it is a natural substance that has the potential to be supportive, if the issues continue, it is recommended that a full evaluation and discussion with a physician take place.

Within the scope of this chapter, we will provide comprehensive information regarding the recommended dosages and duration of usage of Tribulus terrestris. In addition, we will go over recommendations for safe use as well as potential interactions with other medications or supplements in order to supply you with the information you need to make educated choices.

4.5 Known side effects and possible interactions with other substances

Tribulus terrestris may have some adverse effects, and it may also interact with other substances. These side effects and interactions are possible. In the following part, we will discuss the known adverse effects of Tribulus terrestris as well as the potential interactions that it may have with other substances.

Despite the fact that Tribulus terrestris is considered to be a natural material, it is nevertheless possible for it to cause some adverse effects. One of the most well-known adverse effects is discomfort in the gastrointestinal tract, which can manifest as nausea, abdominal pain, and diarrhea. Typically, these adverse effects are not severe and don't last long. Taking Tribulus terrestris with a meal is recommended in order to reduce the amount of pain experienced by the stomach.

Moreover, there is a possibility that certain individuals are susceptible to Tribulus terrestris, which can result in allergic reactions. In the event that allergy symptoms manifest themselves, such as a rash, itching, swelling, or difficulty breathing, the consumption of the substance should be immediately stopped, and a medical professional should be consulted.

You should be aware that Tribulus terrestris has the potential to influence the levels of glucose in your blood. Because of this, individuals who have diabetes should get the advice of their physician prior to consuming Tribulus terrestris and should also periodically monitor their blood glucose levels.

In addition, there is the possibility of interactions with both other medications. Because Tribulus terrestris, for instance, has the potential to reduce blood pressure, it is important to exercise caution if you are already using antihypertensive medication. It is strongly suggested that you consult with a medical professional or a pharmacist before beginning treatment with Tribulus terrestris, particularly if you are already using other medications.

However, it is essential to keep in mind that Tribulus terrestris may have an effect on the control of hormones. Before beginning treatment with Tribulus terrestris, individuals who are already receiving hormone therapy or who have hormonal abnormalities should seek the advice of a medical professional.

In this chapter, we will explore the potential interactions between Tribulus terrestris and other substances, as well as provide specific information regarding the commonly seen adverse effects of this plant. Before beginning to use Tribulus terrestris, it is strongly recommended that you get the advice of a medical professional or an expert, particularly if you are already taking medication or have a history of health issues. We want to ensure that you are able to make decisions based on accurate information and that you always keep your health in mind.

Chapter 5: Ashwagandha

5.1 Traditional use of Ashwagandha in Ayurvedic medicine

Withania somnifera, more commonly referred to as ashwagandha, is a herb that has been utilized in the practice of traditional Ayurvedic medicine for a considerable amount of time. In this chapter, we will discuss the traditional applications of ashwagandha as well as the significance of this herb for the vitality of men.

In Ayurvedic medicine, ashwagandha is referred to as rasayana, which implies that it is believed to have a renewing impact on the body. The immune system is strengthened, energy and vitality are increased, and general well-being is promoted by its use, as it has been used traditionally. It is considered an adaptogenic herb, which means that it can assist improve sexual function and increase libido. Ashwagandha is also regarded to be beneficial to male virility.

Ashwagandha is traditionally used in a manner that is consistent with the principles of Ayurveda, which is an ancient Indian medicinal technique. In the field of Ayurvedic medicine, ashwagandha is frequently regarded as a tonic for males, as it has the potential to assist in promoting sexual health and restoring equilibrium to the body. Ashwagandha is said to have the ability to facilitate the alleviation of stress, the enhancement of endurance, and the enhancement of physical performance, all of which can have a beneficial impact on male virility.

Ingestion of Ashwagandha powder, production of Ashwagandha tea, and the use of Ashwagandha extracts are all examples of traditional applications of Ashwagandha. Other applications include the use of Ashwagandha extracts. The precise dosage and method of application may differ from person to person, depending on the requirements of the individual and the advice of an Ayurvedic physician.

In spite of the fact that the traditional application of ashwagandha is founded on a great deal of experience and folklore, it is essential to keep in mind that it is not necessarily supported by scientific evidence. In spite of this, a number of research have demonstrated encouraging findings about the possible effects of ashwagandha on male virility. Before beginning to use ashwagandha, it is recommended that you wait for additional research discoveries and, if required, seek the advice of a medical professional.

A comprehensive examination of the traditional application of Ashwagandha in Ayurvedic medicine, as well as the prospective significance of this herb for male vitality, will be presented in this chapter. For the purpose of providing you with a thorough information foundation, we shall examine both the old mythology and the most recent scientific findings related to the topic.

5.2 Potential to increase sexual performance

Ashwagandha, a plant that has been used for traditional Ayurvedic treatment for a very long time, is frequently related with improving sexual performance. In this section, we will investigate the possibility of ashwagandha to improve sexual function in a more in-depth manner.

There have been a number of research that have claimed that ashwagandha may have beneficial impacts on female sexual health and performance. There is a widespread belief that ashwagandha has the potential to boost sexual satisfaction, improve sexual stamina, and stimulate libido to a greater extent. Ashwagandha is known to have adaptogenic characteristics, which are known to help relieve stress and increase general well-being. This is the reason why this is the case.

It has been demonstrated in a number of studies that ashwagandha has the ability to boost the generation of nitric oxide, which in turn can enhance blood flow and contribute to a more robust erection process. Additionally, it is believed that ashwagandha has the ability to regulate hormone levels in the body, particularly the levels of testosterone, which is an essential hormone for both sexual and reproductive function.

When it comes to sexual performance, it is essential to keep in mind that the effects of ashwagandha can differ from person to person. Some men may feel a significant improvement in their sexual function and desire, while others may only notice slight changes in their sexual function and desire. There is a possibility that the benefits of ashwagandha are also influenced by other elements, such as one's lifestyle, nutrition, and overall health.

There is no universally accepted method for determining the ideal dosage of ashwagandha for the purpose of improving sexual performance. It is strongly suggested that the dosage guidelines for the product be adhered to, or that the counsel of a physician or other knowledgeable individual be sought. There are a few different ways that ashwagandha can be consumed, including powder, capsules, or extracts; the dosage needs to be adjusted according to the product.

Ashwagandha should not be considered the only cure to sexual issues; rather, it should be considered a supportive strategy to boost sexual performance. This is an essential point to keep in mind. In order to obtain the best possible outcomes, it is possible that you may need to take a holistic strategy that incorporates a healthy lifestyle, a balanced diet, and possibly even additional treatments.

We are going to take a comprehensive look at the potential of Ashwagandha to improve sexual function in this chapter. The purpose of this article is to provide you with a comprehensive overview of this natural ingredient by discussing scientific findings, testimonies, and possible methods of application. When trying to obtain the greatest possible results, it is essential to establish expectations that are grounded in reality and to take into account the unique characteristics of each individual.

5.3 Effects on stress reduction and general well-being

Not only is ashwagandha recognized for its potential impact on sexual performance, but it is also valued for its capacity to alleviate stress and enhance overall well-being. We are going to investigate the impact of ashwagandha on the decrease of stress and the overall well-being of individuals in this part.

Ashwagandha is classified as an adaptogen, which indicates that it has the ability to assist the body in adjusting to environments that are stressful and in preserving overall equilibrium. Ashwagandha is said to have a relaxing impact on the nervous system and can reduce the production of stress hormones like cortisol. This phenomenon is supported by scientific research. Because of this, tension can be alleviated, anxiety can be reduced, and an inner balance can be promoted.

In addition to having an effect on hormone levels, stress can also have an adverse effect on overall well-being, which can have a detrimental impact on sexual function. As a result of its ability to alleviate stress, ashwagandha has the potential to indirectly enhance sexual function. Increasing sexual desire, improving erectile function, and improving general sexual well-being are all possible outcomes of lessening the effects of stress and anxiety.

In addition, there is a possibility that ashwagandha has further beneficial impacts on one's overall health. There is a commonly held belief that it has the potential to boost one's energy levels, improve mental clarity, and enhance physical endurance. Improving one's overall well-being and enhancing one's sense of vigor and enthusiasm for life are both possible outcomes of this.

Depending on the specific requirements of the individual, the dosage of ashwagandha that is recommended to help stress reduction and general well-being may vary. It is advised that the dosage instructions on the product label be followed, or at the very least, that you seek the counsel of a certified physician or other expert. It is possible to consume ashwagandha in the form of capsules, powder, or extracts; the precise dosage may be determined by the concentration of the substance.

Take notice that ashwagandha should be regarded as a supplement and not as a substitute for leading a healthy lifestyle. This is an essential point to point out. When it comes to achieving best effects, it may be beneficial to practice various stress-reduction tactics in addition to taking ashwagandha. Some of these techniques include relaxation exercises, meditation, and maintaining a balanced diet.

In this chapter, we will take a comprehensive look at the effects that Ashwagandha has on the alleviation of stress and the general well-being of individuals. For the purpose of providing you with a thorough grasp of this natural material, we will discuss both the traditional applications and the scientific findings. Through the incorporation of Ashwagandha into a healthy lifestyle, one may experience an enhanced sense of well-being as well as improvements in their sexual health.

5.4 Different dosage forms and dosage recommendations

There are many different dosage forms of ashwagandha, and it is essential to take the appropriate amount in order to attain the best possible outcomes. In this section, we will discuss the various dosage forms of Ashwagandha as well as the dosages that are advised for use.

There are three different forms of ashwagandha that can be purchased: capsules, powder, and extracts. The choice of dosage form is frequently determined by personal preferences and the specific requirements of the individual. Each dosage form has its own set of benefits and drawbacks.

One of the most common and easy ways to consume ashwagandha is through capsules. These capsules come with a pre-determined amount of the extract and are simple to consume by mixing with water. Because the recommendations for dosage differ from product to product, it is essential to read and adhere to the directions that are printed on the product label. In general, it is recommended that one consume between 600 and 1200 milligrams of ashwagandha in the form of capsules on a regular basis.

There is a wide variety of applications for ashwagandha powder. Blending it into smoothies, juices, or other beverages is a possibility. In general, the recommended dosage for ashwagandha powder is between one and two teaspoons per day, which is equivalent to around two to four grams. To ensure that the active components are distributed evenly throughout the powder, it is essential to thoroughly mix the powder.

Ashwagandha extracts are concentrated forms of ashwagandha that often contain a greater quantity of the active component than they do in their natural form. Because the dosage recommendations for ashwagandha extracts might change depending on the concentration, it is essential to adhere to the guidelines provided by the manufacturer with regard to dosage. There is a common range of 250 to 500 milligrams for the daily dose that is advised.

It is essential to keep in mind that the dosages of ashwagandha that are prescribed are basic guidelines that can be altered according to the specific needs of each individual. When beginning treatment, it is advisable to begin with a lesser dosage and gradually raise it as required. In particular, if you are already taking other medications or have concerns about your health, it is recommended that you read the dosage guidelines that are included on the product label or seek the opinion of a suitable physician or other knowledgeable individual.

It is also possible for the length of ashwagandha use to change. There are individuals who consume ashwagandha on a consistent basis for an extended period of time, while there are others who simply use it temporarily to support particular objectives. For the purpose of assessing the effects of ashwagandha and making any required adjustments, it is recommended that you keep track of your use of this herb over a period of many weeks or months.

In this chapter, we have discussed the various dose forms of Ashwagandha as well as the dosages that are advised for use. To achieve the best possible outcomes, it is essential to adhere to the prescribed dosage. Always refer to the dose guidelines that are printed on the product label, or seek the advice of a trained professional, in order to determine the appropriate dosage for your specific requirements.

5.5 Safety profile and possible limitations

The safety of ashwagandha is usually considered to be satisfactory, particularly when it is consumed in the dosages that are commonly suggested. There have been very few instances of major adverse effects that have been related with the consumption of ashwagandha. Nevertheless, it is essential to take into consideration a few possible restrictions.

Ashwagandha may elicit a moderate sedative effect, which is one of its potential adverse effects. Due to this, some people may experience feelings of drowsiness or seclusion. When beginning treatment with ashwagandha, it is advisable to begin with a lesser dosage and watch how the body reacts to the supplement. It is recommended that the dosage be reduced or the time of consumption be modified in the event that drowsiness or sleepiness occurs. This is done to prevent any potential interference with everyday activities.

More than that, there is some evidence to suggest that ashwagandha can reduce the amount of sugar in the blood. This may be relevant for individuals who suffer from hypoglycemia or diabetes because it has the potential to result in an extra decrease in blood sugar levels. Ashwagandha should only be consumed by individuals who are under the supervision of a medical professional, since this is the recommendation.

An allergic reaction to ashwagandha has also been reported, however it is quite uncommon for such reactions to occur. It is recommended that ashwagandha not be used by anyone who are known to have allergies to plants belonging to the nightshade family, which includes ashwagandha.

On top of that, there is a possibility that ashwagandha will interact negatively with some drugs. Before beginning to take ashwagandha, it is strongly suggested that persons who are already taking medication check with their physician or pharmacist to explore the possibility of any interactions that may occur.

When considering the use of Ashwagandha, pregnant women and women who are breastfeeding should exercise caution and check with their physician before beginning to take the supplement. There is a lack of knowledge regarding the safety of ashwagandha during pregnancy and lactation; therefore, it is recommended that due diligence be taken.

In conclusion, ashwagandha is typically safe to consume when it is taken in the dosages that are suggested. Nevertheless, persons who are taking medications, have certain health conditions, or are

allergic to certain substances should exercise caution
and seek the advice of a skilled physician or pharmacist before beginning to consume ashwagandha.
To guarantee that the usage of ashwagandha is both
safe and effective, it is essential to take into account
the safety profile of the herb and to pay attention to
any potential limits.

Chapter 6: Horny Goat Weed (Epimedium)

6.1 History and legends around Horny Goat Weed

A plant with a complex history and countless legends surrounding its use, Horny Goat Weed, also known as Epimedium, is a plant that is also known by its scientific name. It is believed that the origins of Horny Goat Weed can be traced back to Chinese mythology and modern medicine.

Horny Goat Weed has been used for ages in Chinese tradition to boost male virility and increase sexual desire. This practice dates back through the centuries. The name of the plant is claimed to originate from a folklore in which shepherds noted that goats who consumed Horny Goat Weed exhibited heightened sexual behavior. This led to the plant's moniker. As a result of this observation, the hypothesis that Horny Goat Weed could have comparable effects on human beings was developed.

Furthermore, the plant has a long history of application in Chinese medicine, where it has been used to treat sexual dysfunction as well as other health issues. It is well known for its ability to strengthen the yin and yang energy systems, as well as for its tonic effect on the kidneys. Traditional Chinese medicine frequently employs the usage of Horny Goat Weed in conjunction with other herbs in order to amplify the benefits of the herb and to foster a state of equilibrium within the body.

This plant is a fascinating component of natural means of improving male vitality because of the legends and lengthy history of utilizing it. Horny Goat Weed is made up of different parts. The use of it has persisted over the centuries and continues to be extremely popular even in the present day.

In the following sections, we will take a more in-depth look at the potential advantages that Horny Goat Weed may have for male virility and sexual performance. In order to provide you with a full review of the effects, applications, and potential limitations of this unique plant, we will present information from the scientific community.

6.2 Active ingredients and their effects on male virility

The herb known as Horny Goat Weed, also known as Epimedium, is thought to contain a number of different bioactive chemicals, which are thought to be responsible for its potential impacts on male virility and sexual performance. The chemical known as icariin, which is regarded to be the primary active component of Horny Goat Weed, is one of these compounds.

Icariin is a flavonoid that is categorized as a phytoestrogen and has a structure that is comparable to that of testosterone, which is responsible for male sexual activity. By enhancing the generation of nitric oxide, icariin is thought to increase blood circulation. This is thought to be accomplished by its interaction with enzymes found within the body. This, in turn, can cause blood vessels to widen and increase the amount of blood that flows to the vaginal region, which can enhance both the erection and the sexual performance of the individual.

Furthermore, there are additional possible consequences that are related with the use of Horny Goat Weed. It has been hypothesized that the plant possesses anti-inflammatory characteristics and has the ability to bring the body's hormones into equilibrium. There is a possibility that this will have a beneficial impact on libido, sexual endurance, and overall well-being.

This is a crucial point to keep in mind because additional research is required to determine the precise mechanisms and effects of Horny Goat Weed on male virility. Further human clinical research are required to prove the efficacy and safety of Horny Goat Weed on male virility. This is despite the fact that there is promising evidence from laboratory and animal studies as well as traditional usage of the herb.

In the following sections, we will provide you with a full overview of the current scientific evidence and go into greater detail on the various benefits and applications of Horny Goat Weed. When it comes to the use of Horny Goat Weed, we will also go over the various restrictions and safety measures that should be taken.

6.3 Possible applications and recommended dosages

Epimedium, often known as Horny Goat Weed, can be utilized in a variety of forms, such as extracts, capsules, powders, and tinctures. Considering that every one of these dosage forms comes with its own set of benefits and drawbacks, it is up to you to select the one that caters to your requirements and preferences the most effectively.

When taking Horny Goat Weed, it is essential to adhere to the dosages that are prescribed in order to achieve the best potential outcomes and reduce the likelihood of experiencing any unwanted effects. There is a possibility that the precise dosage will change based on the product and the concentration of the active component; thus, it is recommended that the directions provided by the manufacturer or the package insert be carefully studied.

A daily dose of between 500 and 1000 milligrams is advised for the majority of extracts derived from horny goat weed. This dose can be broken up into multiple smaller doses that can be taken individually in order to guarantee that the active ingredient is distributed evenly throughout the day. The quantities that are indicated for use with Horny Goat Weed capsules or powder can vary from 500 mg to 2000 mg per day, depending on the concentration of the active ingredient that is included in the specific product.

It is essential to keep in mind that Horny Goat Weed may not start working right away, and that consistent use over a longer period of time may be necessary in order to reach the desired outcomes. It is possible that the effect will differ from one individual to the next, and it may take a few weeks before the full benefits are experienced.

Before beginning to take Horny Goat Weed or any other dietary supplement, it is strongly recommended that you consult with your physician or pharmacist. This is especially important if you are currently taking other medications or have any pre-existing health concerns. With the help of your physician, you will be able to receive personalized dosage recommendations that take into account the potential for interactions with other substances.

It is important to keep in mind that Horny Goat Weed is a dietary supplement and should not be used as a replacement for a healthy lifestyle and a diet that is already well-balanced. In order to promote your male vitality, it is essential to take into consideration other areas of your lifestyle, such as engaging in regular physical activity, getting sufficient sleep, learning how to manage stress, and maintaining a good diet.

As a means of assisting you in making an educated choice, we will offer you with comprehensive information regarding the potential adverse effects and precautions that you should take into consideration when taking Horny Goat Weed in the following sections.

6.4 Known side effects and possible drug interactions

There is a possibility that using Horny Goat Weed could result in certain adverse effects; however, these symptoms are often uncommon and moderate. There is a possibility of experiencing slight pain in the gastrointestinal tract, which may manifest as nausea, diarrhea, or indigestion. In extremely unusual instances, you can also have symptoms such as headaches, dizziness, or skin rashes. It is absolutely necessary to be aware of the fact that every organism may react differently, and that the adverse consequences may differ from one individual to the next.

In addition, it is essential to be aware of the potential interactions that may occur between Horny Goat Weed and other drugs. Horny goat weed has the potential to alter the effects of a number of pharmaceuticals, particularly those that thin the blood, those that treat diabetes, those that lower blood pressure, and particularly those that treat depression. For this reason, it is highly recommended that you consult with your physician or pharmacist prior to consuming Horny Goat Weed, particularly if you are currently taking additional medicine.

When you use Horny Goat Weed in conjunction with your prescriptions, your physician or pharmacist can assist you in determining whether or not it is safe to do so and identifying any potential interactions that may occur. They are also able to provide you with information on how to properly dose the medication in order to reduce the possibility of adverse effects.

Furthermore, it is essential to take into consideration specific categories of individuals who could not be good candidates for the consumption of horny goat weed. Individuals that fall under this category include those who suffer from specific medical illnesses, such as cardiovascular disease, low blood pressure, liver disease, or hormone issues. It is also recommended that women who are pregnant or breastfeeding abstain from using horny goats.

You should check for quality and safety in Horny Goat Weed, just as you would with any other dietary supplement. Make sure to get items from reputable manufacturers and seek for the label that indicates the product's tested quality and purity. Be sure to thoroughly read the product information and adhere to the dosing recommendations.

In the event that you have any symptoms or side effects that are not typical while using Horny Goat Weed, you should immediately immediately cease using it and seek medical attention.

To provide you with a full perspective, we will examine the legal implications of Horny Goat Weed products as well as the availability of these items in the next chapters.

6.5 Available products and quality standards

It is possible to get Horny Goat Weed in a number of different forms, such as capsules, tablets, extracts, and powder. A person's preferences and requirements should guide their selection of the appropriate dose form. Extracts and powders are more adaptable and can be utilized in a variety of applications, including beverages and food. Capsules and tablets provide a convenient and accurate method of dosing.

In the process of purchasing items containing Horny Goat Weed, it is essential to pay attention to the quality and purity of the product. You should look for products that come from reputed producers who adhere to sound production methods and carry out quality control tests. Certifications such as ISO 9001 and GMP (Good Manufacturing Practice) can serve as an indicator of the quality of a product. Make sure you are purchasing a product of great quality by carefully reading both the product information and the reviews left by other customers.

At the same time, the concentration of active substances in the products is another significant issue to consider. One of the compounds found in Horny Goat Weed is called icariin, and it is widely believed to be the primary active component responsible for the virility-enhancing effects of this plant. Be on the lookout for items that include a large amount of icariin, as this can interfere with the effectiveness of the product.

Finding out where the plants that are being used came from is another thing that should be done. A variety of places, including China and other parts of Asia, are responsible for the cultivation of horny goat weed. Better quality can be achieved by using products that are grown in a sustainable manner and do not contain any harmful residues.

In order to attain the best results possible, it is essential that the dosages be followed exactly as they are recommended. Depending on the substance and the concentration of the active ingredient, the precise dosage may change from one instance to another. In order to establish the appropriate dosage for your specific requirements, you should either consult a physician or a pharmacist, or follow the directions that are printed on the product's box.

Taking dietary supplements such as Horny Goat Weed is not a replacement for maintaining a healthy lifestyle and eating a balanced diet. This is an important point to keep in mind. It is also essential for general vitality and virility to have a nutritious diet, engage in physical activity, and get a proper amount of sleep.

Within the following chapters, we will investigate various more natural compounds that are beneficial to male vitality in order to present you with a full range of options and knowledge.

Chapter 7: Saw palmetto

7.1 Origin and distribution of saw palmetto

The saw palmetto, also known as Serenoa repens in the scientific community, is a kind of plant that is primarily indigenous to North America. It can be found growing in the subtropical parts of the southeastern United States, mainly in the state of Florida and neighboring states around the Gulf Coast. A number of other names, such as dwarf palm, sabal palm, and Serenoa dwarf palm, are also used to refer to saw palmetto.

The name "saw palm" refers to this particular variety of palm, which is distinguished by its bushy look and distinctively saw-shaped leaves. It is possible for the plant to grow to a height of up to three meters and to produce thick colonies from which many stems emerge. The saw palmetto tree produces fruits that are tiny and dark in color. These fruits contain seeds that are sought after for their medicinal qualities.

Throughout the course of history, saw palmetto has played a significant role in the traditional medical practices of the indigenous peoples of North America. Native American communities utilized the fruits of the saw palmetto tree as a remedy for a wide range of diseases, including issues that were associated with the reproductive system and the urinary tract. Saw palmetto was also utilized by Native American tribal traditional healers in order to alleviate inflammation and improve general health.

In modern times, saw palmetto is mostly valued for its potential to improve virility and its capacity to maintain the health of the prostate. Saw palmetto has been shown to be useful in alleviating the symptoms of benign prostate enlargement, which is often referred to as benign prostatic hyperplasia (BPH). This has been proved by a number of scientific research. It is believed that the active chemicals found in the fruits of saw palmetto, such as phytosterols and flavonoids, have the ability to reduce inflammation and have an effect on the balance of hormones.

Saw palmetto can be purchased in a number of different forms, including extracts, capsules, and tablets, among others. The choice of dose form is determined by the individual's preferences as well as their specific requirements. Extracts are frequently sold in highly concentrated forms of the active component, but capsules and tablets offer a handy and accurate method of measurement for administering the medication.

When selecting goods containing saw palmetto, it is essential to pay attention to the quality and purity of its ingredients. When shopping for items, look for those that come from reputable producers who adhere to quality control procedures and follow excellent production methods. In order to guarantee that you are purchasing a product of superior quality, it is important to thoroughly read the product description and become familiar with any relevant certifications, such as GMP (Good Manufacturing Practice).

When it comes to saw palmetto products, the suggested dosage may change depending on the concentration of the active ingredient as well as the specific requirements of each individual. When trying to establish the appropriate dosage, it is best to either follow the directions that are printed on the product's box or seek the opinion of a medical professional or a pharmacist.

In the coming chapters, we will examine additional natural compounds that are beneficial to male vitality in order to give you with a broad variety of options and knowledge.

7.2 Link between saw palmetto and prostate health

Saw palmetto (Serenoa repens) has established itself as a natural solution to support prostate health. Numerous scientific studies have confirmed the positive effects of saw palmetto on the symptoms of benign prostate enlargement, also known as benign prostatic hyperplasia (BPH).

Saw palmetto contains a variety of bioactive compounds such as phytosterols, flavonoids and fatty acids, which are known for their anti-inflammatory properties. These active compounds can help regulate prostate growth and reduce inflammation in the area. By inhibiting the production of dihydrotestosterone (DHT), a hormone associated with BPH, they support healthy prostate function.

The positive effect of saw palmetto on prostate health is manifested in the reduction of BPH symptoms such as frequent urination, nighttime urination, difficulty urinating, and weakened urinary stream strength. Studies have shown that taking saw palmetto extracts can lead to significant improvement in these symptoms, increasing overall well-being and quality of life in men with BPH.

The exact mode of action of saw palmetto on the prostate is not yet fully understood, but it is believed that the plant's bioactive compounds affect several mechanisms, including inhibition of the enzyme 5-alpha reductase, which is responsible for converting testosterone to DHT.

When using saw palmetto to support prostate health, it is important to follow the correct dosage. When it comes to the product and the concentration of the active substances, the recommended dosages may differ from one another. It is advisable to read the manufacturer's instructions carefully and, if necessary, seek advice from a doctor or pharmacist to determine the optimal dosage for your individual needs.

It is important to note that taking saw palmetto alone may not be sufficient to treat serious prostate conditions. If symptoms persist or are severe, it is advisable to consult a doctor for an accurate diagnosis and appropriate medical treatment.

Saw palmetto can be purchased in a number of different forms, including extracts, capsules, and tablets, among others. Choose high-quality products from trusted manufacturers to ensure optimal efficacy and safety. Look for certifications such as GMP (Good Manufacturing Practice), which indicate good manufacturing practices.

In the following chapters, we will explore other natural male vitality substances to provide you with a comprehensive selection of options and information.

7.3 Influence on hormone balance and sexual function

There is a possibility that saw palmetto, also known as Serenoa repens, can influence the hormonal equilibrium and sexual function of men. Research is being conducted to determine whether or whether this substance has the potential to influence the levels of the male hormone testosterone, and consequently, to promote sexual health and function.

It has been discovered that saw palmetto has the ability to inhibit specific enzymes, in particular 5-alpha reductase, which is the enzyme that is accountable for the transformation of testosterone into dihydrotestosterone (DHT). Saw palmetto has the ability to control testosterone levels in the body and prevent an excessive conversion to DHT by blocking an enzyme that is responsible for this process. The hormonal balance may be improved as a result of this effect, which also support good sexual function.

It is essential for men to have adequate levels of testosterone in order to maintain their sexual health and overall well-being. Testosterone is an important hormone that plays a role in the control of sexual function, libido, erections, and the creation of sperm. Saw palmetto can assist improve sexual function and performance for a number of reasons, including the fact that it helps maintain hormone health.

Additionally, there have been a few studies that have been carried out that point to the potential role that saw palmetto could have in the treatment of erectile dysfunction treatment. However, the precise mechanisms by which saw palmetto impacts sexual function are not completely understood, and for this reason, additional research is required to better understand the interactions between these two factors.

Saw palmetto may not be adequate on its own to treat sexual dysfunction or other significant sexual disorders. This is an important point to keep in mind. It is recommended that you consult a medical professional in order to have a thorough evaluation and individualized treatment if you continue to experience difficulties with your sexual function.

In accordance with the specific requirements of each individual, the recommended dosage and duration of Saw Palmetto administration may differ. It is strongly suggested that you carefully follow the instructions provided by the manufacturer and seek the advice of a medical professional or a pharmacist if necessary in order to determine the appropriate dosage for your particular circumstance.

In the next chapters, we will investigate additional natural male vitality compounds in order to present you with a broad range of options and knowledge.

7.4 Correct dosage and duration of use

When it comes to getting ideal results in sustaining male vitality, it is essential to utilize Saw Palmetto

(Serenoa repens) for the appropriate dosage and for the appropriate amount of time. It is essential to adhere to the dosage guidelines that have been prescribed, and if appropriate, to seek the advice of a physician or a pharmacist.

It is possible for the recommended dosage of Saw Palmetto to change based on the product and the concentration available. The instructions that are printed on the label of each product should be read carefully and followed to the letter. In some instances, the recommended dosage is expressed in milligrams, while in others, it is suggested that a particular quantity of capsules or tablets be used on a daily basis. In order to determine an individual's level of tolerance, it is recommended to gradually increase the dosage.

It is also possible for the length of Saw Palmetto use to change. Furthermore, in order to make the most of the long-term benefits, it is recommended that you continue taking it for a longer period of time. Several studies have demonstrated that the optimum outcomes can be obtained after a period of time that is either several weeks or months of consistent use. On the other hand, it is essential to take into account the specific unique requirements and responses of the body.

Due to the fact that natural supplements can require some time to reach their full potential, it is recommended that you exercise patience when taking Saw Palmetto. Because it is necessary to conduct an accurate assessment of its efficacy, it is recommended that its utilization be maintained for a period of at least four to six weeks. In the event that it is required, it may be beneficial to check with a natural health professional or a physician on a regular basis in order to adjust the dosage and period of usage accordingly.

Saw palmetto is a dietary supplement, and as such, it should not be used as a replacement for a healthy lifestyle and a balanced diet. It is vital to know that saw palmetto is regarded nutritional supplement. If you want to boost male vitality in a holistic manner, it is recommended that you also pay attention to maintaining a good diet, engaging in physical activity, getting enough sleep, and managing stress.

In the next chapters, we will investigate additional natural male vitality compounds in order to present you with a broad range of options and knowledge.

7.5 Safety profile and possible contraindications

Extensive research has been conducted to determine whether or not saw palmetto, also known as Serenoa repens, is safe to use as a dietary supplement for the purpose of enhancing male vitality. Saw palmetto is generally believed to be well tolerated and exhibits a limited number of positive side effects. On the other hand, it is essential to take into consideration any potential contraindications and precautions.

It has been noticed that the use of saw palmetto does not generally result in any substantial adverse effects in the majority of individuals. On occasion, however, gastrointestinal symptoms such as nausea, vomiting, or diarrhea may manifest themselves. There have been isolated instances of allergic responses being recorded. If you experience or continue to experience these symptoms, you should discontinue the usage of Saw Palmetto and seek the advice of a medical professional.

There are a few conditions that are known to be incompatible with the usage of saw palmetto. Avoiding Saw Palmetto is recommended for people who have a history of allergic reactions to other members of the Arecaceae family, including Saw Palmetto.

Before using Saw Palmetto, it is recommended that individuals under the age of 18 years old, women who are pregnant or breastfeeding, and women who are pregnant or nursing get the counsel of a medical professional.

Additionally, it is essential to take into consideration the possibility of interactions with other medications. Saw palmetto has the potential to potentially alter the way in which certain medications work, particularly those that are based on hormones, such as hormone replacement therapy or contraceptives. Before beginning to use saw palmetto, it is extremely important to consult with a medical professional or a pharmacist, particularly if you are also on other medications.

Saw palmetto is usually considered to be safe and is well tolerated by most people. It is important to take into account any potential contraindications as well as the specific circumstances of each individual. In situations when there is a lack of clarity or specific health concerns, it is recommended to seek the opinion of a specialist. When it comes to natural chemicals, every body is distinct and may react in a different way. Due to the fact that tolerance can vary from person to person, it is essential to pay attention to how your body reacts to the substance and make adjustments or stop using it as required.

In the following chapter, we will focus on a different natural ingredient that has been shown to boost male vitality. We will also offer you with extensive information and suggestions regarding this substance.

Chapter 8: L-Arginine

8.1 Function and importance of L-arginine in the body

One of the necessary amino acids, L-arginine, is responsible for a number of crucial functions throughout the body. This substance plays a role in a number of different biological processes and is of particular significance for the vitality of men.

The generation of nitric oxide (NO) is one of the primary tasks that L-arginine is responsible for. A messenger that assists in the relaxation of blood arteries is called nitric oxide. Consequently, this enables improved blood flow, which includes improved blood supply to the vaginal region. Through its ability to enhance blood flow, L-Arginine has the potential to enhance sexual performance and virility.

In addition to this, L-arginine is involved in the process of maintaining the equilibrium of hormones. There is a possibility that it will stimulate the release of growth hormones, which would then have an effect on libido and sexual performance. Furthermore, L-arginine is a precursor to endogenous chemicals like creatine and proline, which play a significant role in the creation of energy and the metabolism of cells.

It has also been shown that L-arginine can help reduce stress. Through the activation of the nitric oxide pathway, it has the potential to make relaxation more effective and to improve general well-being. This may have a beneficial impact on sexual performance as well as the overall health and well-being of sexuality.

Due to the fact that L-arginine is very important for male vitality, it has become a very popular nutritional supplement. It is frequently made available in the form of L-arginine preparations that are simple to use through oral consumption. Recommendations for dosage change depending on the individual's requirements and current state of health. It is recommendable to adhere to the dosages that are indicated and to seek the counsel of a professional if it is required.

The fact that L-Arginine is not appropriate for everyone is an essential point to keep in mind. Prior to beginning L-Arginine supplementation, individuals who suffer from certain health issues, such as heart disease or low blood pressure, should consult a primary care physician. Additionally, it has the potential to interact with some drugs, including those used to treat virility issues and substances that are used to treat hypertension. For this reason, it is essential to see a medical professional before beginning to use L-arginine, particularly if you are already on other drugs.

In general, L-arginine has the potential to improve male vitality by promoting blood circulation, maintaining hormone balance, and lowering stress levels. Nevertheless, it is essential to take into account people's specific requirements and health concerns. Over the course of the following chapter, we will investigate yet another natural chemical that has been shown to enhance male vitality, and we will also supply you with extensive information and suggestions.

8.2 Effects on blood flow and sexual performance

L-Arginine, which is a natural supplement that boosts male vitality, has the potential to have a substantial impact on blood flow and sexual production. Because of its capacity to generate nitric oxide (NO), it assists in the relaxation of blood vessels, which eventually leads to an increase in blood flow throughout the body, particularly in the genital region.

There is a strong correlation between increased blood flow and a healthy erection as well as excellent sexual function. L-Arginine is able to widen blood vessels by activating the nitric oxide signaling pathway. This results in an increase in blood flow, which in turn enables an erection that is both more powerful and more long-lasting. This has the potential to result in enhanced sexual performance as well as higher satisfaction for the guy and his partner during sexual encounters.

L-arginine may also be helpful in the treatment of erectile dysfunction (ED), which is another condition being treated. According to a number of studies, consuming L-arginine can alleviate some of the symptoms of erectile dysfunction (ED), including the difficulty to keep an erection going. Because of its capacity to enhance blood flow to the penis and to support the function of erectile tissue, L-arginine is responsible for this development.

L-Arginine dosage varies from person to person based on their specific requirements and the state of their health. It is strongly suggested that the dosage guidelines provided by the manufacturer be adhered to, or that expert medical advice be sought. For most people, the recommended daily dosage is between 2 and 3 grams. In order to achieve the best possible outcomes, it is essential to consume L-Arginine on a consistent basis over an extended length of time.

When using L-arginine, it is important to take into consideration the potential adverse effects as well as reactions with other medications. L-arginine is generally well accepted; but, in extremely unusual instances, gastrointestinal problems such as nausea, diarrhea, or abdominal pain may be experienced by the individual. There is also the possibility that it will interact with some medications, particularly those that are meant to treat virility issues and hypertension medications. Because of this, it is essential to seek the advice of a medical professional prior to beginning treatment with L-Arginine, particularly if you are also on other medications.

Increasing blood flow and sexual performance can be accomplished in a natural way with the help of L-

Arginine. It has the potential to improve general well-being and sexual satisfaction, in addition to being an effective treatment for erectile dysfunction. L-arginine has the potential to be an important component of a holistic approach to improving male vitality, particularly when it is combined with a healthy lifestyle and a food that is evenly distributed. Another natural substance that has been shown to have beneficial effects on male virility will be the subject of our discussion in the following chapter, and we will supply you with extensive information regarding this substance.

8.3 Different forms of application and dosage recommendations

L-arginine, a naturally occurring molecule that has been shown to boost male vitality, is available in a variety of applications to cater to the specific requirements of each man. L-arginine can be consumed in a variety of forms, such as by the consumption of powders, supplements, or meals that are rich in L-arginine.

Tablets and capsules are the two forms that dietary supplements that contain L-arginine can be found in. Because the amount of L-arginine that is contained in these dosage forms is mentioned on the label, dosing with them is both convenient and accurate. When taking the capsules or pills, it is advisable to take them with an adequate amount of water and to follow the dosage recommendations provided by the manufacturer.

L-arginine can also be consumed in powder form, which is an additional option. Simply dissolving the powder in water or juice and drinking it is all that is required. This enables adjustable dosage, as the quantity of L-arginine can be varied according to the requirements of the patient. To ensure that the L-arginine is distributed evenly throughout the powder, it is essential to thoroughly mix the powder.

Moreover, there are meals that are naturally abundant in L-arginine, which is another benefit. These include, for instance, meat and poultry, legumes, nuts, seeds, and other similar foods. It is possible to enhance your levels of L-arginine in a natural way by include these foods in your diet. It is important to note, however, that the amount of L-arginine found in foods is typically lower than the amount found in supplements or powders; hence, it may be challenging to consume sufficient amounts.

L-arginine dosage varies from person to person based on their specific requirements and their current condition of health. It is strongly suggested that the dosage guidelines provided by the manufacturer be adhered to, or that expert medical advice be sought. For most people, the recommended daily dosage is between 2 and 3 grams. In order to attain the best possible outcomes, it is essential to take L-arginine on a consistent basis for an extended period of time.

To lessen the likelihood of experiencing pain in the gastrointestinal tract, it is recommended that L-arginine be consumed in conjunction with a meal. Because carbohydrates are known to stimulate the generation of nitric oxide, the use of L-arginine in conjunction with carbohydrates has the potential to even further improve the effect.

When consuming L-arginine, it is essential to take into consideration the unique tolerance of each individual. L-arginine is generally well accepted; but, in extremely unusual instances, gastrointestinal problems such as nausea, diarrhea, or abdominal pain may be experienced by the individual. Before beginning treatment with L-arginine, it is important to seek the advice of a medical professional in the event that such complaints arise or in the event that preexisting health issues are present.

All things considered, L-arginine can be applied in a number of different ways, giving you the opportunity to select the method that is most suitable for you. When taken on a consistent basis, L-arginine can assist boost male vitality and sexual performance. This can be accomplished by the consumption of powders, supplements, or natural foods. Another natural substance that has been shown to have beneficial effects on male virility will be the subject of our discussion in the following chapter, and we will supply you with extensive information regarding this substance.

8.4 Side effects and possible interactions with other substances

The consumption of L-arginine for the purpose of enhancing male vitality is typically well tolerated. Nevertheless, there is a possibility that adverse effects could develop in extremely rare instances. Some of the potential adverse effects include symptoms that affect the gastrointestinal tract, such as nausea, diarrhea, or stomach pain. In most cases, these symptoms are not severe and go away on their own as the body becomes accustomed to the consumption of L-Arginine. To lessen the likelihood of experiencing pain in the gastrointestinal tract, it is recommended that L-Arginine be consumed in conjunction with a meal.

L-arginine has the potential to temporarily lower blood pressure, which is an important fact to keep in mind. As a result, people who have low blood pressure or who are already on medications that lower blood pressure ought to exercise caution and seek the advice of a medical professional before beginning to use L-Arginine. In a similar vein, persons who are already taking drugs that thin the blood should consult a physician before beginning to use L-Arginine because L-Arginine has the potential to increase the effects of blood coloring.

When persons with known heart disease or other significant health concerns are considering the use of L-arginine, it is recommended that they discuss the usage of the supplement with a physician. In certain instances, it may be necessary to monitor the amount of L-arginine that is consumed, or alternative therapeutic approaches may be taken into consideration.

In addition, individuals who are afflicted with genital herpes or other herpes-related conditions ought to exercise caution because L-arginine has the potential to enhance the activity of the herpes virus. When this occurs, it is strongly suggested that you seek medical advice before beginning to take L-Arginine.

It is essential to discuss the possibility of interactions with other medications or supplements that you are currently taking with your primary care healthcare provider. L-arginine has the potential to influence the way certain drugs work, including those that treat hypertension, those that contain nitrates, and those that are used to increase sexual performance. In order to minimize unintended consequences, it is of the utmost importance to give careful consideration to the possibility of interactions.

However, it is important to remember that the information that is presented here is of a general nature and is not meant to serve as a replacement for the advise of a qualified medical practitioner. Taking L-Arginine may cause a variety of responses from individuals because of their individuality. Before beginning to take L-Arginine, it is strongly suggested that you seek the opinion of a medical professional in order to receive tailored guidance and to discuss any potential risks or concerns.

Within the following chapter, we will investigate yet another natural chemical that has been shown to have beneficial benefits on the vitality of men.

8.5 Restrictions on use for persons with certain medical conditions

Despite the fact that L-Arginine has the ability to provide numerous advantages for male vitality, there are certain medical issues that call for particular precautions or may require the use of the supplement to be restricted. Before taking L-Arginine, individuals who suffer from any of the following medical disorders should discuss the matter with their primary care physician:

- Heart disease: In individuals with pre-existing heart disease, including congestive heart failure, coronary artery disease, or cardiac arrhythmias, use of L-arginine may have cardiovascular effects. Medical consultation is important to evaluate the safety and tolerability of L-Arginine in such cases.

- Hypertension: L-arginine may temporarily lower blood pressure. Individuals with hypertension (high blood pressure) should monitor their blood pressure regularly and discuss the use of L-arginine with their physician to determine optimal dosages and tolerability.
- Kidney or liver disease: Individuals with kidney or liver disease should exercise caution as L-arginine is metabolized by the kidneys and liver. It may be necessary to adjust dosage or consider alternative treatment options. Medical advice is essential in such cases.
- Diabetes: L-arginine may affect blood glucose levels. Individuals with diabetes should closely monitor their blood glucose levels and discuss the use of L-arginine with their physician to consider possible effects on blood glucose levels.
- Pregnancy and lactation: The use of L-arginine during pregnancy or lactation should be discussed with a physician, since the effects on the fetus or the breastfed baby have not yet been adequately studied.

Note that the material presented here is of a general character and does not constitute particular medical advice. It is essential that you are aware of this fact. Because of the fact that every person is different, their reactions to L-Arginine may vary. It is therefore recommended that an individual contact with a physician or other health care expert in order to clarify any potential hazards or concerns and to evaluate the tolerance of L-Arginine in relation to the individual's current state of health.

In the following chapter, we will investigate yet another natural element that is an essential component of male vitality on a significant level.

Chapter 9: Zinc

9.1 Role of zinc in male virility and reproductive functions

Zinc is a trace element that is vital to the body and has a significant part in the reproductive and virility processes of males. It can be found in a variety of tissues throughout the body, including the testes, the prostate, and the seminal vesicles, where it is found in substantial quantities. Zinc plays a role in a wide variety of biological processes that are essential for the vitality and sexual health of men.

A sufficient supply of zinc is essential for the creation of testosterone, which is the principal hormone responsible for male sexual activity. In addition to its role in the regulation of sexual processes and sperm production, testosterone is also an important regulator of libido. Zinc plays a role in the process of converting testosterone into its active form, and as a result, it aids to the preservation of a healthy hormonal equilibrium.

In addition to this, zinc has a role in the production of DNA, the division of cells, and the renewal of tissues. When it comes to spermatogenesis, which is the process by which sperm are formed, this is especially important. In order to maintain the integrity, motility, and quantity of sperm, it is essential to have a sufficient supply of zinc.

A lack of zinc has been linked to a number of negative effects on male reproductive function, including a decrease in the quality of sperm, according to a number of pieces of research. Consequently, a sufficient consumption of zinc can contribute to the enhancement of male fertility as well as overall sexual health.

Zinc can be obtained from a variety of sources, including foods and supplements, according to the requirements of health. There are a lot of foods that are high in zinc, including oysters, cattle, chicken, eggs, nuts, and seeds. Zinc demands can be met by the use of supplements, which can be a handy choice, particularly in situations where food consumption is insufficient.

The daily zinc consumption that is suggested varies depending on the individual's age and gender. The use of approximately 11 milligrams of zinc per day is recommended for adult males. However, it is essential to take into account the specific requirements of each individual and alter the dosage accordingly. As a result of the potential for adverse consequences associated with zinc consumption, it is important to avoid exceeding the amount that is prescribed.

People who are taking certain medications or who have specific medical conditions should contact with a physician before using zinc supplements. This is because there is a possibility that zinc supplements could interfere with other medications or cause complications.

In the following chapter, we will investigate yet another plant-based chemical that has the potential to enhance male vitality.

9.2 Optimal zinc intake and sources in the diet

It is essential to consume an adequate amount of zinc in order to acquire the potential health benefits that this trace element may offer. A person's age, gender, and specific requirements all play a role in determining the optimal zinc consumption. An consumption of approximately 11 milligrams of zinc per day is suggested for adult males. When determining the appropriate dosage, it is essential to take into account the specific requirements of each individual.

Zinc requirements can be satisfied by consuming a diet that is both well-balanced and abundant in foods that contain zinc. Among the many natural sources of zinc that are great are:

- Oysters: Oysters are one of the best sources of zinc. They contain high amounts of zinc and at the same time provide valuable proteins and other nutrients.
- Beef: Beef is a good source of zinc. Choose lean beef such as beef tenderloin or lean ground beef to reduce fat content.
- Poultry: Chicken and turkey meat also contain zinc. Opt for lean poultry meat and remove the skin to reduce the fat content.
- Eggs: Eggs are not only rich in protein, but also a source of zinc. You can use them in various dishes or prepare them as omelettes or scrambled eggs.

- Nuts and seeds: Almonds, walnuts, pumpkin seeds and sesame seeds contain zinc. They can be eaten as a snack, added to cereals or salads, or consumed in the form of nut butter.
- Legumes: Lentils, beans and chickpeas are not only a good source of protein, but also rich in zinc. You can use them in soups, stews or as a side dish with meals.

In addition, certain cereals and grain products, such as oatmeal and goods made from whole grains, are also sources of zinc. To ensure that you are getting a wide range of minerals, including zinc, it is essential to consume a diet that is diversified.

If the amount of zinc that is consumed through food is insufficient or if there are particular requirements, dietary supplements might be a viable choice. However, before beginning to use supplements, it is recommended to see a medical professional in order to discuss the appropriate dosage as well as any potential interactions with other medications.

The consumption of an adequate amount of zinc, in conjunction with a diet that is well-balanced, can assist promote male virility and reproductive capabilities. In the following chapter, we will discuss yet another natural component that plays a crucial role in maintaining testosterone levels.

9.3 Effects of zinc deficiency on sexual health.

There is some evidence that a zinc shortage might have a detrimental effect on sexual health and virility. Both the generation of sex hormones like testosterone and the normal functioning of reproductive organs are dependent on zinc, which plays a crucial role in both of these processes. It is possible for low zinc levels to cause a reduction in testosterone production, which in turn can lead to sexual dysfunction and a diminished desire to engage in sexual activity.

In addition, zinc shortage might have an impact on the production of sperm as well as their quality. The process of spermatogenesis, which is the formation of sperm, is dependent on zinc, which also plays a role in the production of healthy sperm. An insufficient amount of zinc can result in a reduction in the number of sperm, a reduction in the motility of sperm, and an impairment in the capacity to fertilize.

Zinc deficiency can also have an effect on immunological function, which can result in an increased risk of genitourinary infections. In turn, infections can have an impact on sexual health and lead to symptoms such as pain or inflammation to manifest themselves.

When trying to avoid these adverse effects, it is essential to ensure that adequate amounts of zinc are maintained. A nutritious diet that includes foods that are high in zinc can assist in meeting zinc requirements. Individuals who are at a higher risk for zinc deficiency, such as vegetarians, vegans, or those with specific medical conditions, may want to plan a conscious inclusion of zinc-rich foods in their diet or consider dietary supplements in conjunction with a physician. This applies to both vegetarians and vegans.

It is essential to keep in mind that maintaining a healthy zinc level is essential, but that consuming an excessive amount of zinc should be avoided.

Additionally, there is the potential for zinc consumption to have adverse impacts on one's health. For this reason, it is essential to adhere to the dosages that are recommended and to seek the opinion of a specialist if it is required.

In the tenth chapter, we will investigate yet another natural element that is essential for the vitality of men and has the potential to have beneficial impacts on sexual health.

9.4 Overdose and potential side effects

The consumption of zinc in excessive amounts can result in unfavorable side effects. Excessive consumption of zinc supplements is not encouraged, despite the fact that zinc is essential for maintaining good health. The gastrointestinal tract can be affected by zinc overdose, which can result in symptoms such as nausea, vomiting, diarrhea, and stomach pain.

An excessive consumption of zinc can also result in a reduction in the body's ability to absorb copper. In the body, zinc and copper are in competition with one another for the same transport mechanisms. Consuming a high amount of zinc can cause the body to absorb less copper, which can result in a severe lack of copper in the body. Copper deficiency, on the other hand, can result in a variety of health issues, including anemia, neurological abnormalities, and reduced immunological function.

It is essential to take zinc supplements in accordance with the specified dosage, and it is not acceptable to take more than the daily dose that suggested. A person's age, gender, and unique requirements all play a role in determining the necessary zinc consumption. If you want to make sure that you are taking the appropriate amount of zinc, it is recommended that you follow the dose instructions that are printed on the product label or seek the counsel of a nutritionist or a physician.

In addition, it is essential to keep in mind that zinc supplements have the potential to interact with other medications or supplements when taken together. Antibiotics, diuretics, penicillamine, and some antacids are all potential medications that could interact with this medication. Therefore, if you are already taking other prescriptions, it is recommended that you consult a physician in order to avoid any potential conflicts between the medications.

In the tenth chapter, we will investigate yet another natural element that is essential for the vitality of men and has the potential to have beneficial impacts on sexual health.

9.5 Advice on supplementation and use of zinc preparations

In the event that you are considering using zinc supplements, it is highly recommended that you consult with a trained nutrition expert or a medical professional before making the decision. These professionals are able to conduct an individual evaluation and offer recommendations that are tailored to the specific requirements and conditions of each individual.

When using zinc supplements, it is essential to ensure that the dosages are adequate and that you take into account the specific zinc requirements of each individual. One's age, gender, current state of health, and particular objectives can all have an impact on the dosage. To establish the appropriate dosage to satisfy the requirements of each individual, a skilled specialist can be of assistance.

Tablets, capsules, powders, and liquids are some of the different forms that zinc supplements can be found in now available. The benefits and drawbacks of each kind are distinct from one another. Personal tastes and specific life situations should be taken into consideration when selecting the appropriate shape. The directions that are printed on the product label should be read carefully, and the dosage that is prescribed should be adhered to.

In addition, it is essential to keep in mind that zinc supplements are typically better tolerated when they are consumed in conjunction with a meal. You may experience less discomfort in your stomach as a result of this.

It is also important to note that zinc supplements should not be considered a replacement for a diet that is well-balanced. It is recommended that the primary source of zinc be a diet that is both nutritious and varied, and that is abundant in foods that contain zinc, such as meat, fish, nuts, seeds, and whole grains. As a means of assisting in the maintenance of zinc levels that are appropriately balanced, supplementation with zinc supplements should be considered.

Last but not least, it is essential to undergo routine examinations in order to guarantee that zinc supplementation has the desired effect and does not have any unfavorable consequences on one's health. If one experiences any adverse effects or is unsure about the treatment, they should seek medical attention as soon as possible.

Chapter 10: Ginkgo biloba

10.1 Botanical characteristics and historical use of Ginkgo biloba

The Ginkgo biloba tree is well-known for the distinctive botanical properties it possesses as well as its extensive history of application in traditional medicine. The ginkgo biloba tree is distinguished by its leaves that are fashioned like fans and by its seeds that are unique. Due to the fact that it is the sole member of its genus to have survived and has a history that spans several million years, it is considered a living fossil.

Since ancient times, Ginkgo biloba has been utilized in the traditional medical practices of a number of different civilizations, particularly in Chinese medicine. For the treatment of a wide range of health issues, including the enhancement of brain function and blood circulation, it has been utilized.

Ginkgo biloba has been used throughout history for a variety of purposes, including its function as an aphrodisiac and its ability to promote masculine vitality. As a result of its ability to boost blood circulation and blood flow to the male reproductive organs, ginkgo biloba is thought to be able to contribute to an increase in sexual function.

Currently, ginkgo biloba can be purchased in the form of herbal medicines and dietary supplements. Extracts from the leaves of the Ginkgo biloba tree are used in these products. These extracts are standardized to ensure that they contain a specific quantity of active components.

The possible advantages of ginkgo biloba for male virility and sexual health will be discussed in further depth in the following portion of this article.

10.2 Potential to increase blood flow and improve sexual function.

Because of the effects that it has on blood circulation and the flow of blood to the sexual organs, ginkgo biloba has the potential to improve sexual function. By virtue of its capacity to expand blood vessels and increase blood flow, ginkgo biloba has the potential to assist in ensuring that the genital region receives an appropriate amount of blood.

It is essential for optimal sexual function to have appropriate blood flow since this enables an adequate supply of oxygen and nutrients to be delivered to the body. The enhancement of blood flow has the potential to enhance sexual response and pleasure, as well as to produce erections.

It has been demonstrated through research that ginkgo biloba has the ability to expand blood vessels, particularly the microscopic capillaries that supply the vaginal region. This has the potential to result in enhanced sexual stamina as well as better erectile function.

Furthermore, it has been shown that ginkgo biloba possesses antioxidant characteristics, which possess the ability to defend against the damage caused by free radicals. Blood vessels can be damaged by free radicals, which can then lead to a reduction in blood flow. Through its ability to protect blood vessels, ginkgo biloba may contribute to the maintenance of healthy blood vessels and the enhancement of sexual function.

On the other hand, it is essential to keep in mind that the way in which individuals react to ginkgo biloba can differ. It is possible that some individuals will have a significant enhancement in their sexual function and the quality of their erections, while others may experience less significant results. It is recommended that the use of Ginkgo biloba be observed over a prolonged length of time in order to allow for an evaluation of the efficiency of the supplement on an individual level.

In the next part, we will discuss the various ways in which Ginkgo biloba can be applied, as well as the dose recommendations that are recommended for it, in order to obtain the greatest potential outcomes.

10.3 Different dosage forms and dosage recommendations

To guarantee that it is easy to use and provides the best possible results, ginkgo biloba is offered in a number of different dose forms. Tablets, capsules, tinctures, and teas are the most prevalent variations of this substance.

Regarding the selection of a dose form, it is essential to take into account one's particular preferences as well as their individual tolerance. While tinctures allow for quicker absorption into the body, tablets and capsules are more handy and easier to ingest than tinctures. An enjoyable approach to consume Ginkgo biloba as a beverage is through the use of teas.

There is a possibility that the dosage of Ginkgo biloba will change depending on the product and the concentration. In order to attain the greatest possible results and refrain from experiencing any potential adverse effects, it is essential to strictly adhere to the dose recommendations provided by the manufacturer.

It is recommended that individuals take 120-240 milligrams of Ginkgo biloba on a daily basis, with the quantity being split into two or three single doses. If you want to ensure greater tolerance and optimal absorption of the active ingredients, it is recommended that you take it with a meal.

When considering the appropriate dosage, it is essential to keep in mind that it may differ from one person to the next. It is possible that some people will have favorable effects at smaller amounts, while others may require a greater dosage in order to obtain the outcomes they are looking for. It is recommended to begin with a smaller dosage and monitor the effects over a period of time in order to establish the dosage that may be appropriate for the individual.

In order to attain the most favorable outcomes, it is recommended that the consumption of Ginkgo biloba be maintained for an extended length of time. Typically, it takes a few weeks of consistent use before one may experience the full effect of the product.

Before beginning to use Ginkgo biloba, it is recommended to get the advice and suggestions of a qualified medical expert or physician in the event that there is any uncertainty or specific health concerns about the use of this supplement.

To guarantee that the usage of Ginkgo biloba is safe, we will examine the potential adverse effects and safety measures that are linked with the herb in the following section.

10.4 Safety profile and possible contraindications

Generally speaking, ginkgo biloba is well tolerated; but, just like any other supplement, there are certain safety concerns and potential contraindications that should be taken into consideration.

Side effects that are modest and only transient are conceivable in the majority of situations. The occasional occurrence of gastrointestinal symptoms such as nausea, indigestion, or headaches are included in this category. In most cases, these adverse effects are extremely uncommon and frequently fade away on their own once the body has become accustomed to the consumption of Ginkgo biloba powder.

Nevertheless, it is essential to act in accordance with certain precautions. Individuals who are known to have an allergy to Ginkgo biloba or any of its components should refrain from taking it. Furthermore, persons who are scheduled to have surgery or who have a history of bleeding issues should not take ginkgo biloba because it has the potential to induce blood clotting. Additionally, persons who are taking drugs that thin the blood should visit their physician prior to taking ginkgo biloba in order to avoid any potential interactions with the drug.

It is also important to note that there are certain contraindications that should be avoided when using Ginkgo biloba. Both pregnant women and nursing mothers are included in this category since there is insufficient information regarding the safety of Ginkgo biloba for these populations. It is also recommended that people who suffer from epilepsy, severe mental illness, or seizures refrain from taking it since ginkgo biloba has the potential to increase the risk of seizures.

If a person is currently on medicine or has a history of pre-existing medical disorders, it is strongly recommended that they seek the advice of a medical professional before beginning to use ginkgo biloba. In addition to providing tailored guidance, the physician is able to establish whether or not it is safe for a person to use ginkgo biloba.

It is essential to emphasize that dietary supplements, such as ginkgo biloba, should not be seen as a replacement for a healthy lifestyle and a diet that is well-balanced. When it comes to developing male vitality and virility, they ought to be taken into consideration as a component of an all-encompassing strategy.

In order to make an educated selection when selecting supplements, we will examine the many products that include Ginkgo biloba as well as the quality criteria that are associated with those goods in the next chapter.

10.5 State of research and scientific findings

A great number of research have been carried out over the course of the last few decades to study the potential of Ginkgo biloba for improving male vitality and sexual health. A number of fascinating insights into the impacts of this natural chemical are provided by the findings of the scientific research.

According to the available research, Ginkgo biloba has the potential to enhance blood flow, particularly in the region of microcirculation. Increasing the amount of blood that flows to the vaginal region and boosting erections are two ways in which this may have a beneficial impact on sexual function. Individuals who suffer from erectile dysfunction may experience an improvement in their erectile function if they take ginkgo biloba, as demonstrated by a number of studies.

Ginkgo biloba is also being investigated for its potential to decrease inflammation and its antioxidant effects, both of which are now being investigated. The presence of these traits may contribute to the enhancement of overall health and indirectly assist sexual function.

With that being said, it is essential to point out that the research that is now available is inconclusive, and additional research is required in order to comprehend the precise mechanisms and impacts that Ginkgo biloba has on male vitality. Moreover, the quality of the studies and the design of the investigations can vary, which can result in different findings.

In spite of this, a significant number of males have reported that they have experienced beneficial outcomes as a result of taking ginkgo biloba, including enhanced sexual function and an overall sensation of enhanced well-being. However, it is recommended that the consumption of Ginkgo biloba be coordinated with a physician and that careful consideration be given to the selection of high-quality goods.

We will look at some practical recommendations and guidance on how to use ginkgo biloba and other natural ingredients for male vitality in the following chapter. This content is intended to assist you in putting these ideas into practice in your own life.

Chapter 11: Ginger

11.1 Traditional use of ginger as an aphrodisiac agent

Since ancient times, people from many different cultures have recognized the numerous health benefits that ginger, a plant with a fragrant scent, offers. In this chapter, we will discuss the traditional use of ginger as an aphrodisiac, as well as the potential impacts that ginger may have on the energetic state of men.

In many different civilizations all over the world, ginger is regarded as a natural aphrodisiac with sexual properties. Since ancient times, people have been consuming ginger to boost their sexual desire and performance. This practice stretches back to ancient times. In Ayurvedic medicine, ginger is referred to as a "hotter" because it is regarded to be a spice that is warming, which increases blood circulation and offers vitality.

There is a wide variety of potential modes of action that ginger could have on male vitality. Ginger has several benefits, but one of the most important ones is that it improves blood circulation. Having a healthy blood flow is essential for healthy sexual activity because it guarantees that the vaginal region receives a sufficient quantity of blood. An additional benefit of ginger is that it can help reduce inflammation and maintain hormonal balance, all of which can have a favorable impact on sexual health.

It is essential to keep in mind that the traditional use of ginger as an aphrodisiac has not been demonstrated to be in accordance with scientific research. Despite the fact that there is some encouraging evidence from studies conducted on animals and in laboratories, there is still a dearth of more thorough clinical trials that can confirm the precise impact that ginger has on male virility and vitality.

Despite this, a significant number of men have had favorable experiences with ginger in terms of its ability to support their sexual health and performance. As a spice that may be used in food and beverages, ginger can also be consumed as a dietary supplement. Ginger can be included into the diet in a variety of different ways.

Within the following part, we will discuss specific applications and dose recommendations for ginger in order to enhance male vitality. Our goal is to provide you with actionable information and suggestions about how to proceed.

11.2 Influence on blood circulation and sexual health

An increase in blood flow and improved sexual health are two potential benefits of ginger. When it comes to sexual function, having enough blood circulation is essential since it guarantees that the genital region receives the appropriate amount of blood. Certain bioactive chemicals found in ginger, such as gingerol and zingiberene, have the ability to improve blood flow and increase blood flow by dilating blood vessels and increasing blood flow.

Ginger has been found in studies to improve vascular health and blood flow with its ability to stimulate blood flow. The reduction of erection issues and the enhancement of sexual function can be facilitated by increased blood flow. Ginger may also help reduce inflammation in the body, which may potentially have a role in sexual health. In addition, ginger may help reduce this inflammation.

It is essential to keep in mind that the effects of ginger on sexual health might differ from person to person, and that not all men will experience the same outcomes as a result of consuming ginger. In order to keep one's sexual health in good condition, it is essential to commit to a healthy lifestyle that includes engaging in regular physical activity, eating a balanced diet, and avoiding dangerous behaviors such as smoking and drinking an excessive amount of alcohol.

If you want to reap the potential benefits of ginger for your sexual health, there are a few different ways that you may add ginger into your diet. Grate ginger fresh, use it as a spice in dishes and beverages, or take it as a dietary supplement. Ginger can be utilized in all of these ways. The exact dosage is determined by a number of factors, including the method of intake and the individual's specific requirements. It is recommended that the dose instructions on the products be followed, or if necessary, a consultation with a physician or pharmacist should be sought out.

It is our intention to provide you with concrete action steps on how to utilize ginger to enhance your sexual health and virility. In the following part, we will examine the many applications of ginger as well as the dosage recommendations for ginger.

11.3 Forms of application and dosage recommendations

For the purpose of reaping the potential benefits of ginger for sexual health, there are a variety of applications for ginger. The following is a list of techniques and dose recommendations generally used:

- Fresh ginger: Fresh ginger can be peeled and grated to use in food and drinks. You can consume about 1 teaspoon of freshly grated ginger per day to benefit from its beneficial properties. Add the grated ginger to your tea, smoothies or cooked dishes to enhance the flavor.
- Ginger tea: Ginger tea is a popular way to consume ginger. You can thinly slice fresh ginger and pour hot water over it. Let the tea steep for about 5-10 minutes before drinking it. One to two cups of ginger tea per day

may be enough to achieve the desired effects.

- Ginger capsules or preparations: Ginger is also available in the form of capsules or preparations. Dosage recommendations may vary depending on the product. Therefore, read the instructions on the packaging carefully and follow the recommended dosage.

It is essential to keep in mind that the appropriate amount of ginger may differ from person to person depending on their requirements and their level of tolerance. Start with a smaller dosage, and if you do not experience any unpleasant side effects, gradually raise it until you reach the desired level. If you have pre-existing health conditions or are currently taking medication, it is strongly suggested that you adhere to the dosage guidelines that are printed on the products or seek the advice of a physician or pharmacist; this is especially important.

It is important to keep in mind that ginger might not have an instant effect, and that it might be necessary to utilize it consistently over a considerable amount of time in order to obtain favorable outcomes. Ginger may provide significant benefits for sexual health, but in order to gain those benefits, consistency is essential.

We shall examine the safety features of ginger in the following part, as well as analyze the potential adverse effects and contraindications associated with its use.

11.4 Possible side effects and precautions

Ginger is generally believed to be safe when it is consumed in dosages that are adequate. Some individuals, on the other hand, may be hypersensitive to ginger and experience adverse reactions to it. You should be aware of the following potential adverse effects and precautions, which are listed below:

- Stomach discomfort: Some individuals may experience stomach discomfort such as heartburn, acid regurgitation, or upset stomach after consuming ginger. This may occur especially if ginger is taken in large amounts. If you are sensitive to ginger, reduce the dosage or consult a doctor.

- Bleeding risk: Ginger may have a blood thinning effect and increase the risk of bleeding. If you are taking blood-thinning medication or have a bleeding-related condition, it is advisable to consult a physician before using ginger.
- Drug interactions: Ginger may interact with certain medications and affect their effects. For example, ginger may increase the effect of blood-thinning medications. If you regularly take medication, talk to your doctor before using ginger as a dietary supplement.
- Allergic reactions: In rare cases, people may have an allergic reaction to ginger. If you notice symptoms of an allergic reaction such as rash, itching, swelling, or difficulty breathing, stop taking ginger and seek medical attention.
- Pregnancy and lactation: Pregnant women should avoid ginger in large quantities as it may increase the risk of miscarriage. It is recommended to consult a doctor before using ginger during pregnancy or lactation.

When using any kind of dietary supplement, it is essential to take into account different people's tolerance levels and to adhere to the recommended dosage. It is highly recommended that you seek the advice of a medical professional or a pharmacist if you have any questions or concerns, particularly if you are currently taking other medications or have pre-existing health conditions.

With the knowledge that you now possess regarding the possible adverse effects and precautions, you are able to make well-informed decisions and use ginger in a responsible manner as a component of your natural support for male vitality.

11.5 Possible combinations with other natural substances

Ginger can be used in combination with other natural substances to increase male vitality and virility. Here are some potential combinations you can consider:

- Ginseng: The combination of ginger and ginseng is often used to promote sexual performance and increase energy. Both plants have stimulating properties and can complement each other to enhance the effect.

- L-Arginine: Ginger can be combined with L-Arginine to further improve blood flow. L-arginine is an amino acid that promotes the production of nitric oxide in the body, which in turn dilates blood vessels and increases blood flow.
- Tribulus terrestris: This plant is often used to increase testosterone levels and improve sexual function. The combination of ginger and Tribulus terrestris may have synergistic effects and support sexual health.
- Maca: Maca is a root from the Andes and is traditionally used to increase libido and sexual stamina. The combination of ginger and maca can help improve sexual function and energy.

A mixture of natural chemicals can have a variety of impacts on various people, which is something that should be taken into consideration. Due to the fact that every individual's body reacts differently to various drugs, it is recommended to carefully monitor the dosages and, if necessary, seek the advice of a traditional medical practitioner or a natural medicine professional.

It is recommended that before to attempting any combination of natural substances, one should first conduct research on the unique effects and probable interactions that may occur. There is a possibility that certain combinations are not appropriate for everyone, particularly if you have a history of health issues or are currently taking other medications.

It is essential to keep in mind that natural remedies are not miraculous cures, and that a healthy lifestyle, including a balanced diet, adequate exercise, and effective stress management, is similarly essential. The combination of natural ingredients, on the other hand, has the potential to play a supporting function and contribute to the promotion of male vitality.

Chapter 12: Saffron

12.1 Cultural significance and use of saffron as a virility agent

There is a long history of saffron being used as a sexual enhancer, and it has cultural importance. Because of its aphrodisiac properties and its ability to boost sexual energy, saffron has been utilized in a variety of cultures for centuries. Saffron is a highly sought-after ingredient in both culinary and medical applications due to its distinctive characteristics, including its strong red color and flavor.

As a sexual stimulant, saffron can be utilized in a variety of different modes of application. Saffron is traditionally utilized in the form of spices or extracts to enhance sexual function and desire. Both of these applications are common. It is believed that certain compounds found in saffron, such as crocin, have the ability to increase blood flow and stimulate the production of endorphins in the brain, both of which may contribute to increased sexual performance.

The use of saffron in everyday life can also be accomplished through a variety of additional means. To take advantage of the possible benefits that saffron may have for male vitality, for instance, it might be incorporated into beverages such as teas, drinks, or smoothies. In addition, there are nutritional supplements and special preparations available on the market that contain saffron extracts and can be utilized expressly for the purpose of enhancing virility that are available.

When using saffron, it is essential to adhere to the dosage recommendations that have been provided. In order to achieve a potential impact, the quantity of saffron required may vary and is contingent upon a number of factors, including the metabolism and health of the individual. It is strongly suggested that you adhere to the instructions that are printed on the products or the suggestions that are made by a physician or an expert in natural medicine.

In addition, it is essential to keep in mind that saffron is not a wonder medication, and that the outcomes may differ from person to person. There is a possibility that the effects of saffron will differ from person to person. It is recommended that saffron be considered as a component of a healthy lifestyle and balanced diet that also includes physical activity, stress management, and taking sufficient amounts of rest.

In the event that you have any inquiries or issues regarding the utilization of saffron as a sexual enhancer, it is highly recommended that you seek the advice of a recognized naturopath or physician. They are able to offer specific guidance and assistance throughout the process of selecting the appropriate dosage and method of application for saffron.

In general, saffron's potential to enhance male vitality makes it an intriguing alternative to consider. On the other hand, it is essential to have reasonable expectations and to take into account the use of saffron as a component of an all-encompassing strategy for enhancing virility.

12.2 Influence on mood and sexual desire

It has been demonstrated that saffron has an effect on both mood and sexual desire. Several research have been conducted to evaluate the causal relationship between saffron and an improvement in mood. It is believed that specific components of saffron, including as crocin and safranal, have the ability to influence the release of neurotransmitters in the brain, which are responsible for the regulation of mood.

Saffron consumption has been shown to result in elevated levels of serotonin and dopamine, both of which have been shown to have a beneficial impact on one's mood. It is possible that this will result in a general improvement in well-being as well as a reduction in tension and worry. This can lead to an increase in sexual desire and satisfaction, which can be a result of improved mood and lower levels of stress.

It is essential to keep in mind that the effects of saffron on one's psychological state and sexual desire can differ from person to person. A person's reaction to the consumption of saffron may vary from person to person. It is possible that the desired benefits will not be seen for some time. Being patient and keeping a close eye on the consequences on a frequent basis is recommended.

It is possible to use saffron in a variety of different ways in order to enhance one's mood and sexual drive. Taking saffron as a dietary supplement is one approach that can be taken. In addition, there are beverages and teas that include saffron and have the potential to have a beneficial impact on one's mood. At the same time that it has the ability to improve one's mood and sexual drive, saffron may also be used as a spice in the kitchen to enhance the flavor of food.

It is important to note that the recommended dosage of saffron differs from product to product and from person to person. In order to establish the appropriate dosage, it is essential to either follow the directions that are printed on the packaging or seek the advice of a natural health practitioner or a physician.

Additionally, it is important to remember that saffron might not be appropriate for all individuals. It is important for individuals who suffer from certain medical disorders or allergies to seek medical advice before consuming saffron. In addition, there is a possibility of interactions with other available medications. The consideration of potential dangers and safety measures is of utmost importance.

Saffron, in general, has the potential to be a natural alternative that can positively influence mood as well as sexual desire. On the other hand, it is recommended to have reasonable expectations and to take into consideration the use of saffron as a component of an all-encompassing strategy for enhancing male vitality.

12.3 Correct dosage and application methods

In order to attain the best possible outcomes, it is essential to pay close attention to the correct dosage and application methods of saffron. It is essential to adhere to the directions that are printed on the product box or the suggestions that are provided by a natural health expert or a natural health practitioner. To help you determine the appropriate dosage and administration of saffron, here are some general guidelines:

- Food supplements: When saffron is taken in the form of capsules or tablets, the recommended dosage is usually between 15 and 30 mg per day. This dosage may vary depending on the product, so it is important to read and follow the specific instructions.
- Saffron tea: For the preparation of saffron tea, you can infuse about 10 to 15 threads of saffron in hot water. The infusion time is

about 10 to 15 minutes. The tea can then be strained and drunk hot or cold. One cup of saffron tea per day can be considered an appropriate dosage.

- Use as a spice: In cooking, saffron can be used as a spice to enhance the flavor of dishes. It is advisable to use saffron sparingly, as its flavor and aroma are intense. A pinch of saffron threads or a small amount of ground saffron may be sufficient to achieve the desired effect.

If you are going to take saffron, it is essential to think about using it on a consistent basis for an extended period of time. Some people may not see the effects of saffron right away, and it may take a few weeks before they notice the effects that they are looking for. Saffron should be used for an extended period of time, and it is recommended that patience be exercised.

It is essential to keep in mind that saffron is a spice that is of high quality and comes at a high price. Saffron should be purchased from reliable sources in order to guarantee that it is of excellent quality and does not include any impurities. This is the reason why it is recommended to do so.

In addition, saffron should not be considered a replacement for a healthy lifestyle and a diet that encompasses a broad range of foods. It is still essential for male vitality to maintain a balanced diet, engage in regular physical activity, and get an adequate amount of sleep.

It is recommended that you seek the assistance of a natural health practitioner or a physician in the event that you have any queries or uncertainties regarding the appropriate dosage and application of saffron. These individuals are able to provide tailored instruction and suggestions.

Remember that everyone is unique and may react differently to saffron. It is important to listen to your body and be aware of any adverse reactions. If you notice any side effects or allergic reactions, you should stop taking saffron and consult a doctor.

12.4 Safety profile and possible limitations

Generally speaking, saffron is believed to be safe when it is used in the recommended proportions. However, there are a few potential limits and safety considerations that should be taken into consideration:

1. Allergic reactions: Some people may have an allergic reaction to saffron. If you notice an allergic reaction such as rash, itching, swelling, or difficulty breathing, you should stop taking saffron immediately and seek medical attention.
2. Pregnancy and lactation: There is limited information on the use of saffron during pregnancy and lactation. It is recommended to be cautious during these periods and consult a doctor before using saffron.
3. Drug interactions: Saffron may potentially interact with certain medications, especially antidepressants, sedatives, and blood-thinning medications. If you are taking such medications, talk to your doctor before using saffron to avoid potential interactions.
4. Gastrointestinal discomfort: In some cases, high doses of saffron may cause

gastrointestinal symptoms such as nausea, vomiting or diarrhea. It is important to follow the recommended dosage and watch out for possible side effects.

5. Caution with certain medical conditions: Individuals with certain medical conditions such as bleeding disorders, diabetes or hormonal imbalances should consult a physician before using saffron to discuss potential risks.

It is important to note that saffron is not a miracle drug and its effect may vary from person to person. The individual reaction to saffron may depend on various factors such as health, dosage and duration of use.

It is recommended to discuss the use of saffron with a natural health professional or physician, especially if you have specific health concerns or are already taking other medications.

In conclusion, saffron is a natural substance that is considered safe when used properly and in appropriate amounts. Nevertheless, potential risks and individual circumstances should be considered to ensure the best possible use of saffron.

12.5 Recommendations for the purchase and storage of saffron

When purchasing saffron, it is essential to pay close attention to the characteristics of the product, specifically its quality and authenticity. The following are some suggestions that will assist you in purchasing saffron of high quality:

- Choose certified saffron: Look for saffron that comes from a trusted source and has certificates confirming its quality and purity. Certified saffron products often come with a test seal that proves their authenticity.
- Check the appearance: Real saffron consists of dried red threads with an intense aroma. Avoid saffron powder or ground saffron threads, as they may have been stretched with other ingredients. Instead, choose

whole threads that are intact and bright red in color.

- Consider the price: Saffron is a precious spice plant, and genuine saffron has a corresponding price. Be wary of extremely cheap offers, as this may indicate inferior or counterfeit products.
- Prefer organic: Organically grown saffron can be free of pesticides and chemical residues. If possible, choose organic saffron to ensure higher quality and purity.

After purchase, it is important to store saffron properly to maintain its quality and effectiveness. Here are some storage recommendations:

- Dark and cool storage: Store saffron in a cool, dry place away from sunlight and moisture. It is best to use an airtight container to minimize contact with air and moisture.
- Avoid heat sources: Do not store saffron near heat sources such as stove or oven as this may affect the quality.
- Limited shelf life: Saffron loses flavor and color over time. Try to use saffron within 1

to 2 years after purchase to ensure the best quality.

By buying high quality saffron and storing it properly, you can ensure that you get the maximum effect and quality of this natural substance for your male vitality.

Conclusion

Within the pages of this book, we have investigated a wide range of natural compounds that have the ability to enhance sexual health and promote the vitality of men. We have discussed twelve of these chemicals in great detail and explained the affects that each of them has on virility and sexual function in their own separate ways. As a conclusion, we would like to emphasize the most significant findings once more, which are as follows:

- Maca, Tribulus terrestris, ginseng, saw palmetto, L-arginine, zinc, ginkgo biloba, ginger and saffron have been identified as natural substances that can have a positive effect on male virility and sexual performance. They can promote blood circulation, influence hormone balance, increase mood and sexual desire.
- We have presented different application forms and dosage recommendations for each of these substances. It is important to observe the correct dosage and choose the recommended forms of application to achieve optimal results.

- In addition to the positive effects, we have also discussed possible side effects and precautions. Every single substance can have an individual effect on the body, and it is important to consider potential risks and contraindications.
- We would like to emphasize that a balanced diet and a healthy lifestyle are fundamental pillars for good sexual health. The use of natural substances can be a supplement, but it is important to take a holistic approach and pay attention to a healthy lifestyle.
- Finally, we would like to point out that it is always advisable to consult a doctor before taking supplements or changing dietary habits. Each person is individual and it is important to take into account individual needs and medical history.

There is a significant possibility that the natural compounds that have been provided can help boost male virility and sexual health. On the other hand, research in this area is still currently being conducted, and new discoveries may one day result in an even deeper comprehension of these chemicals and their potential applications. In order to take advantage of the most recent discoveries in the scientific community, it is beneficial to continue to monitor advances in this area.

In closing, we would like to stress that the purpose of this book is to serve as a source of knowledge and is not meant to serve as a replacement for the advise of a medical professional. We have high hopes that the knowledge and conclusions contained in this book will assist you in making well-informed judgments and considering the possibility of incorporating natural chemicals into your personal male vitality approach.